What is Aphasia?

Aphasia is a language disorder that affects a person's ability to communicate effectively. It can be caused by a brain injury, such as a stroke or traumatic brain injury, or by a degenerative disease, such as Alzheimer's disease. People with aphasia may have difficulty speaking, understanding speech, reading, and writing.

A workbook for people with aphasia after stroke is a comprehensive resource designed to support individuals who have experienced communication difficulties as a result of a stroke.

If you or someone you know has experienced communication difficulties as a result of a stroke, a workbook for people with aphasia after stroke can be a valuable resource for improving language and communication abilities. Here are a few reasons why you may want to consider purchasing a workbook:

Targeted exercises and activities

A workbook for people with aphasia after stroke contains a range of exercises and activities that are specifically designed to target areas of language and communication that have been impacted by the stroke. These exercises can help to improve word retrieval, sentence construction, and conversational skills, among other things.

Easy to use...

The workbook is designed to be user-friendly and can be used independently or with the guidance of a speech therapist. The exercises and activities are presented in a clear and straightforward manner, making them accessible for anyone who is experiencing communication difficulties.

Personalized goals <3

includes space for setting personalized communication goals and developing strategies for achieving them. This can help to ensure that the exercises and activities in the workbook are tailored to the individual's specific needs and interests.

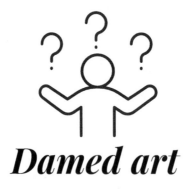

Damed art

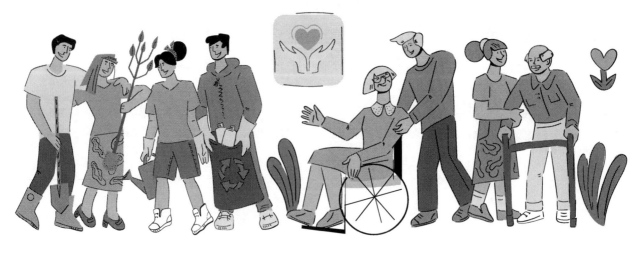

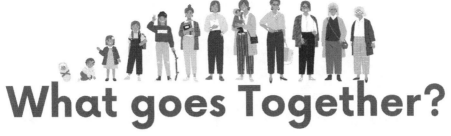

What goes Together?

Match the pictures that belong together.

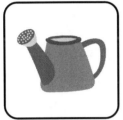   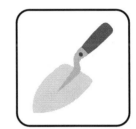

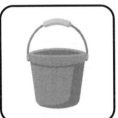   

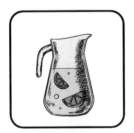   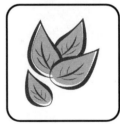

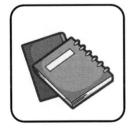 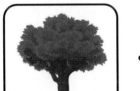   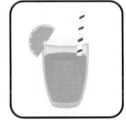

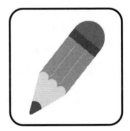

Let us Spell!

Circle the word that is spelled correctly for each picture.

	grass	grasse	gross
	wink	winge	wing
	scisors	scissors	scissore
	earth	aerth	werth
	remute	remote	rimote
	shoes	shoese	shoas
	pilow	pellow	pillow

Z IS FOR...

Follow the guide to trace the letters, then complete the mazes:

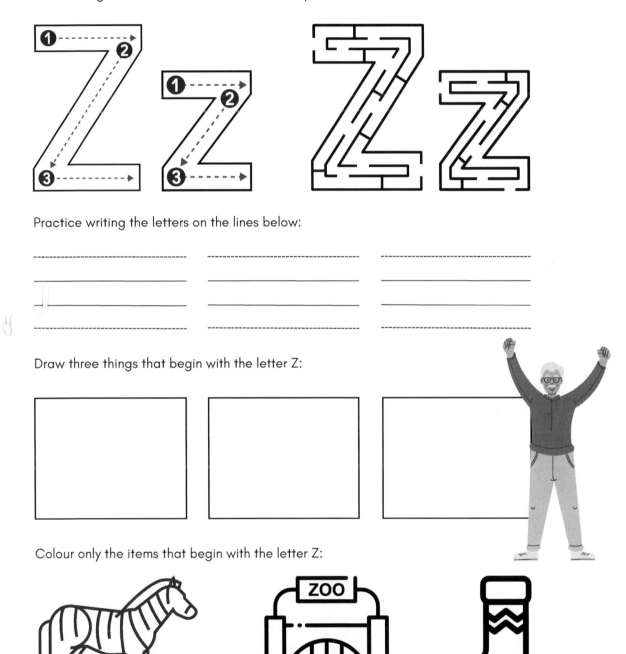

Practice writing the letters on the lines below:

------------------------------   ------------------------------   ------------------------------

_____   _____   _____

------------------------------   ------------------------------   ------------------------------

Draw three things that begin with the letter Z:

Colour only the items that begin with the letter Z:

Fruits

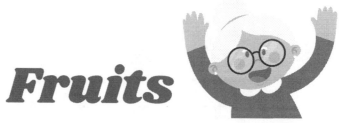

Unscramble the words and write on the blanks.

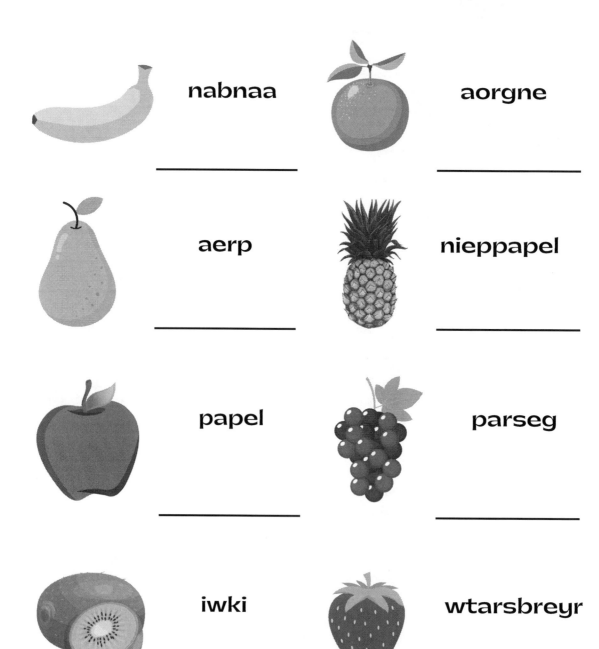

nabnaa

_____

aorgne

_____

aerp

_____

nieppapel

_____

papel

_____

parseg

_____

iwki

_____

wtarsbreyr

_____

O IS FOR...

Follow the guide to trace the letters, then complete the mazes:

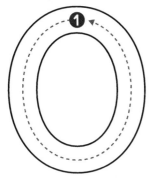 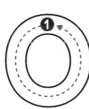 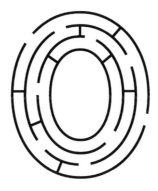 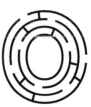

Practice writing the letters on the lines below:

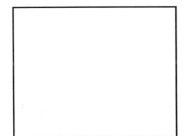 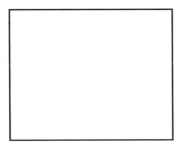 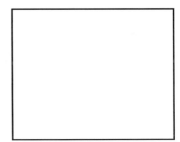

Draw three things that begin with the letter O:

Colour only the items that begin with the letter O:

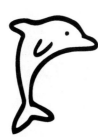  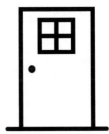

Opposite words

Draw a line to match the word on the left to its opposite.

wet ●   ● slow

hot ●   ● many

long ●   ● hard

fast ●   ● dry

dark ●   ● bright

soft ●   ● short

smooth ●   ● old

young ●   ● rough

few ●   ● cold

INITIAL /F/

Say each word 10x while saying a good "f" sound. Place a checkmark in each circle after saying the sound correctly.

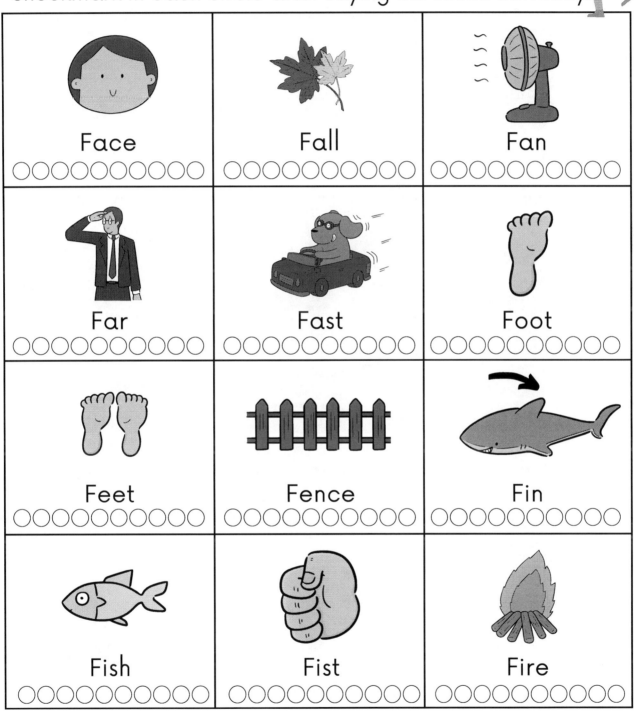

Face	Fall	Fan
○○○○○○○○○○	○○○○○○○○○○	○○○○○○○○○○
Far	Fast	Foot
○○○○○○○○○○	○○○○○○○○○○	○○○○○○○○○○
Feet	Fence	Fin
○○○○○○○○○○	○○○○○○○○○○	○○○○○○○○○○
Fish	Fist	Fire
○○○○○○○○○○	○○○○○○○○○○	○○○○○○○○○○

INITIAL /F/

Say each word 10x while saying a good "f" sound. Place a checkmark in each circle after saying the sound correctly.

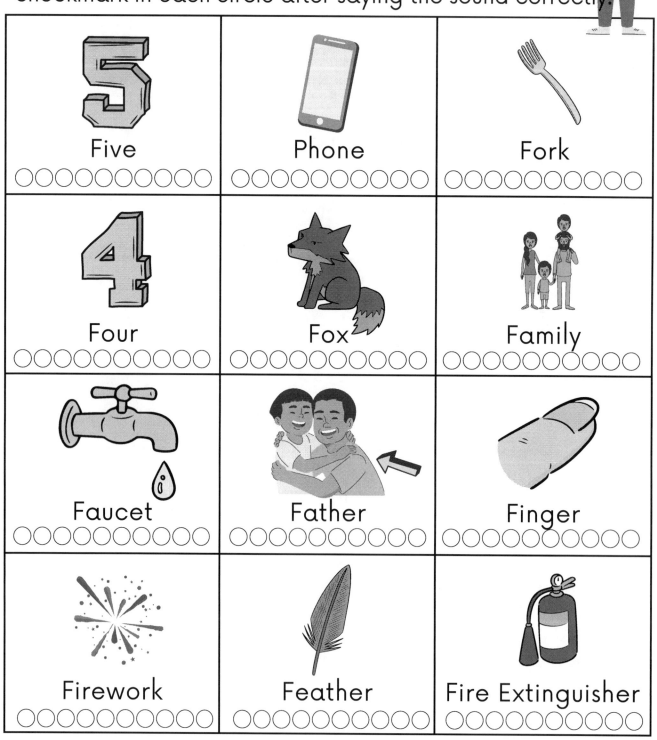

Five	Phone	Fork
OOOOOOOOOO	OOOOOOOOOO	OOOOOOOOOO
Four	Fox	Family
OOOOOOOOOO	OOOOOOOOOO	OOOOOOOOOO
Faucet	Father	Finger
OOOOOOOOOO	OOOOOOOOOO	OOOOOOOOOO
Firework	Feather	Fire Extinguisher
OOOOOOOOOO	OOOOOOOOOO	OOOOOOOOOO

WHAT ? QUESTIONS

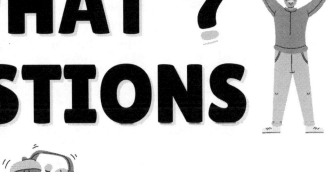

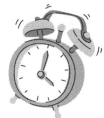

What tells time?

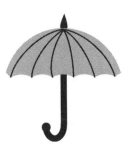

What keeps us dry
in the rain?

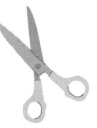

What do we use to
cut paper?

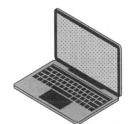

What do you use to
search the internet?

What
questions
ask about a
thing

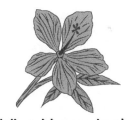

What blooms in the
spring?

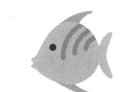

What lives in the ocean?

What do bees make?

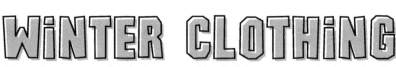

WINTER CLOTHING

Read each clue, then cut out the pictures of the winter clothes below and paste them into the correct box.

What keeps your neck warm?	What keeps your feet warm?	What keeps your head warm?	What keeps your toes warm?
What keeps your body warm?	What keeps your ears warm?	What keeps your fingers warm?	What keeps your hands warm?

- -

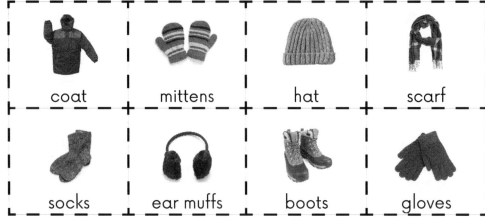

coat	mittens	hat	scarf
socks	ear muffs	boots	gloves

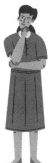

Patterns

Look at the shapes and cross out the one that would come next to complete the pattern.

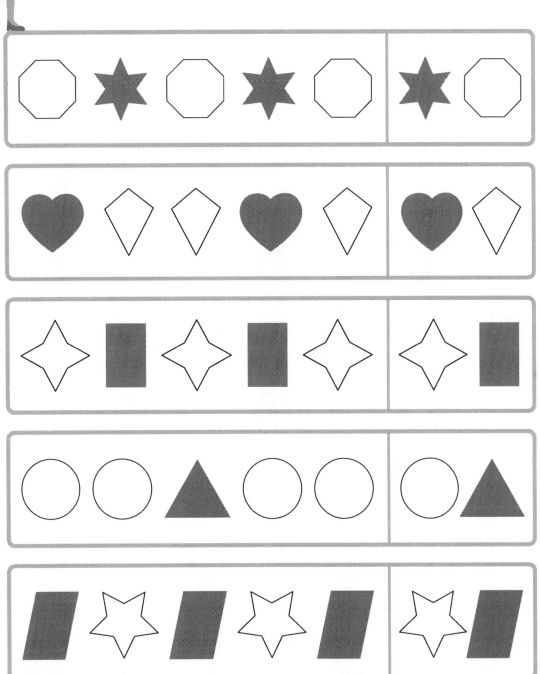

RHYMING WORDS

Match the words that rhyme.

cheese   late

ghost   knees

beg   egg

plate   two

who   glass

class   rat

cat   toast

teach   door

roar   speech

Complete the words with words that rhyme.

1- Would you give me some .... if I said please?

2- Why are you making me beg, I just want an ....

3- It's dinner time. Here's your plate, don't be ....

4- He has got cats which like chasing ....

5- It's science class, don't break any ....

6- If you see a hungry ghost, give it a tasty ....

PREVOCALIC /R/ BINGO

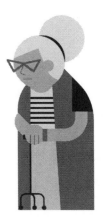

Use a dot marker or bingo chip to mark each word as it is called out. Say each word 10 times with a correct "R" sound to end your turn. If you get five in a row, you win!

Road	Rose	Rug	Ruler	Run
Ring	Roll	Rice	Room	Raft
Race	Radio	FREE SPACE	Red Panda	Rain
Rabbit	Rip	Rake	Rib	Rat
Rainbow	Ram	Rock	Rope	Roof

INITIAL /B/

Say each word 10x while saying a good "b" sound.
Place a checkmark in each circle after saying the
sound correctly.

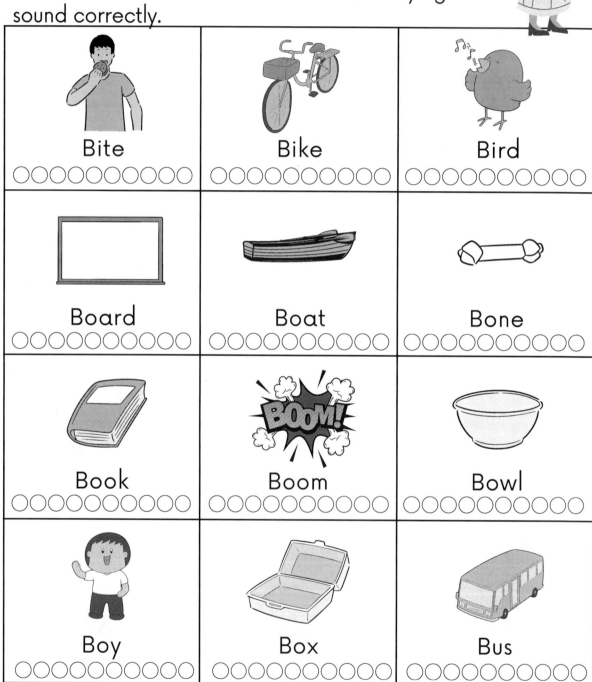

Bite	Bike	Bird
OOOOOOOOOO	OOOOOOOOOO	OOOOOOOOOO
Board	Boat	Bone
OOOOOOOOOO	OOOOOOOOOO	OOOOOOOOOO
Book	Boom	Bowl
OOOOOOOOOO	OOOOOOOOOO	OOOOOOOOOO
Boy	Box	Bus
OOOOOOOOOO	OOOOOOOOOO	OOOOOOOOOO

DESCRIBE THE WINTER WORD

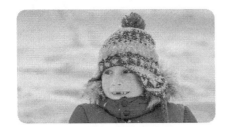

Use the spaces below to describe a winter hat.

group

do

color

where

parts

made of

DESCRIBE THE WINTER WORD

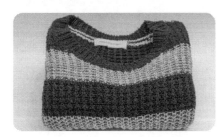

Use the spaces below to describe a sweater.

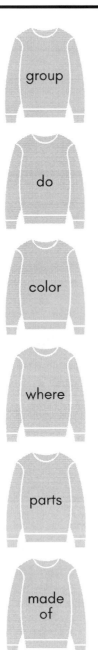

group

do

color

where

parts

made of

_____

_____

_____

_____

_____

_____

_____

_____

_____

_____

_____

_____

DESCRIBE THE WINTER WORD

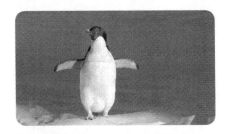

Use the spaces below to describe a penguin.

group

_____

_____

do

_____

_____

color

_____

_____

where

_____

_____

parts

_____

_____

made of

_____

_____

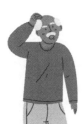

BODY PARTS

The outside of the human body has many different parts that work together.

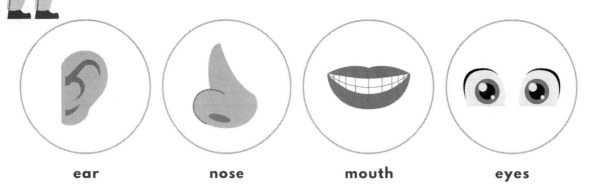

| ear | nose | mouth | eyes |

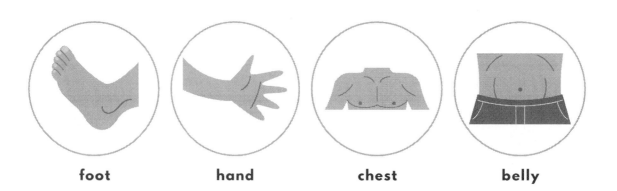

| foot | hand | chest | belly |

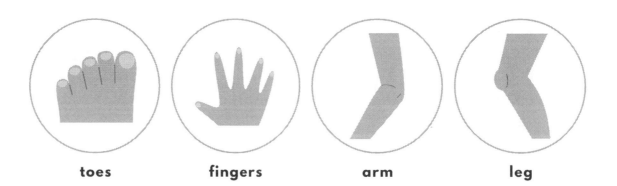

| toes | fingers | arm | leg |

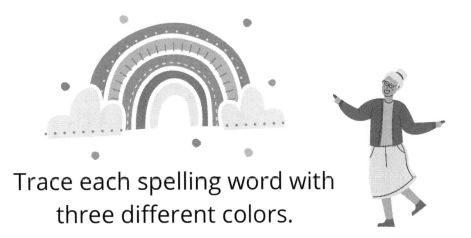

Trace each spelling word with
three different colors.

1. but

2. cut

3. nut

4. shut

5. do

6. slot

7. spot

8. part

9. him

10. his

Days of the Week

Name:_____

Know the names of the seven days in a week.
Copy them on the lines.

1. Sunday

2. Monday

3. Tuesday

4. Wednesday

5. Thursday

6. Friday

7. Saturday

SOFT C SPELLING RULE

Read the words and sort them into soft c words and hard c words by dragging them to the right box.

HARD C	SOFT C

cat   camp   cuddle

pencil   cold   police

city   voice   rice

Let's Count!

Write the missing number on the empty eggs.

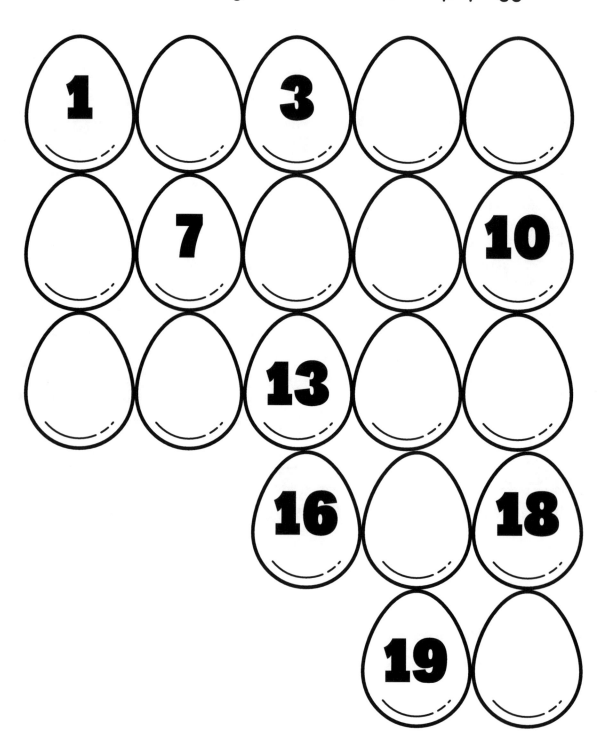

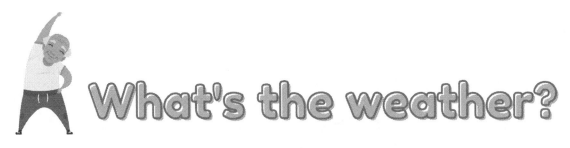

What's the weather?

Direction: Match the weather and the words.

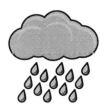 •   • sunny

 •   • cloudy

 •   • stormy

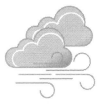 •   • snowy

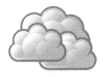 •   • rainy

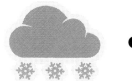 •   • windy

Adding Using Picture

Count the objects, write the number of each and find the sum.

___ + ___ = ___

___ + ___ = ___

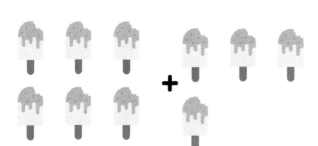

___ + ___ = ___

___ + ___ = ___

___ + ___ = ___

School Objects

Draw a line from each word to the correct picture.

scissor •

•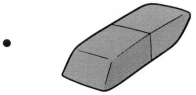

pencil •

•

crayon •

•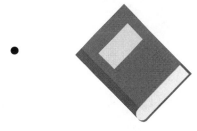

book •

•

eraser •

•

ruler •

•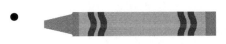

Follow the guide to trace the letters, then complete the mazes:

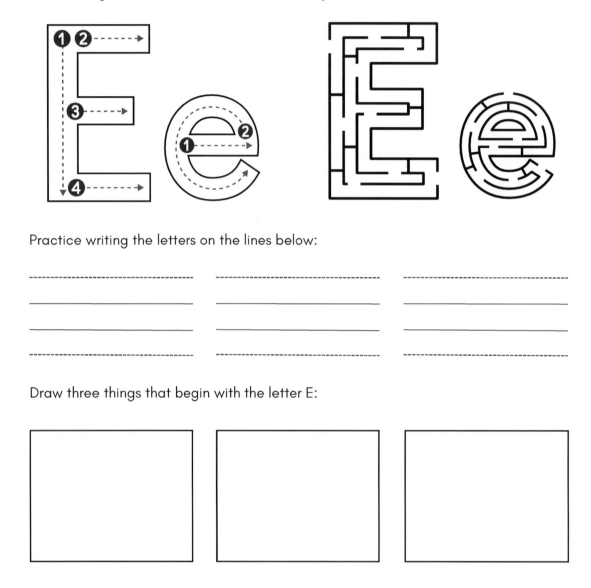

Practice writing the letters on the lines below:

---------------------------------   ---------------------------------   ---------------------------------

_____   _____   _____

_____   _____   _____

---------------------------------   ---------------------------------   ---------------------------------

Draw three things that begin with the letter E:

Colour only the items that begin with the letter E:

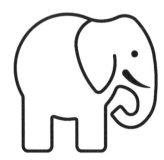

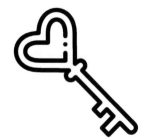

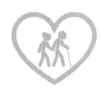

Write the parts of the house. Choose from the box.

garage	bedroom	bathroom
kitchen	living room	dining room

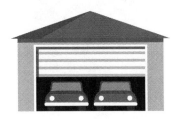

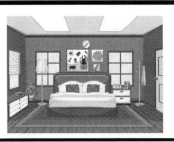

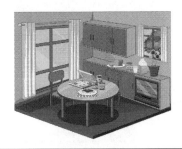

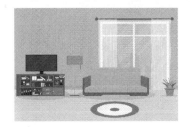

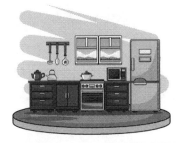

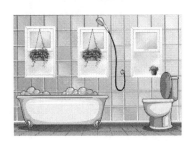

Living and Non-living Things

Classify living and non-living things. Write L for

Living things and NL for Non-living things.

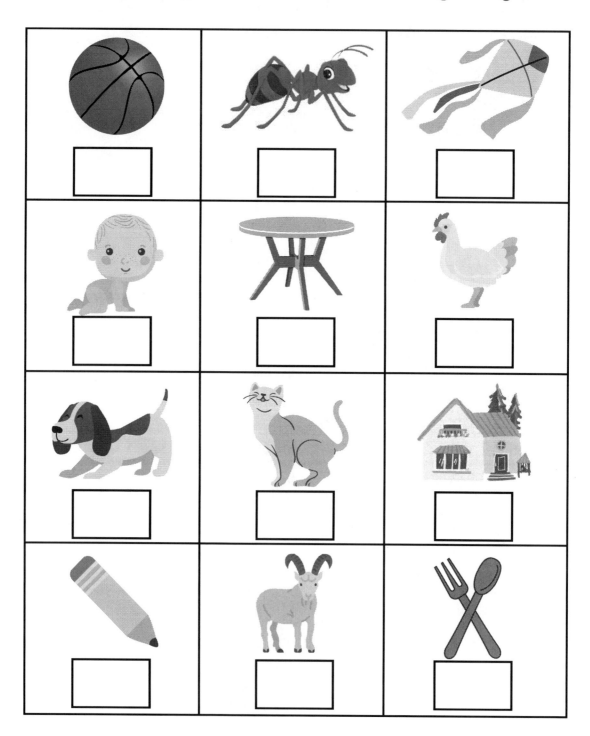

Days of the Week

Cut and paste the days to complete the days of the week.

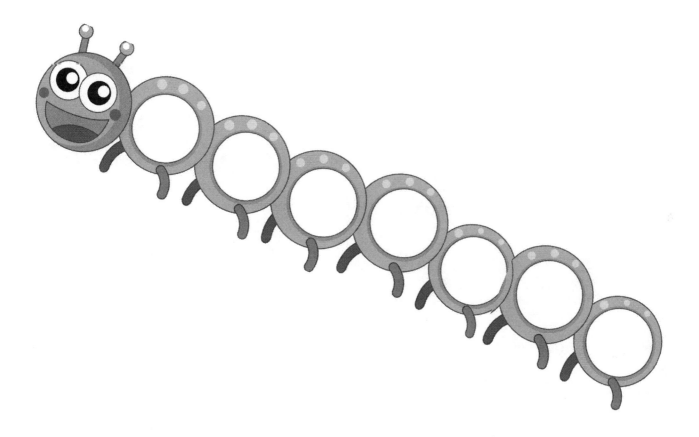

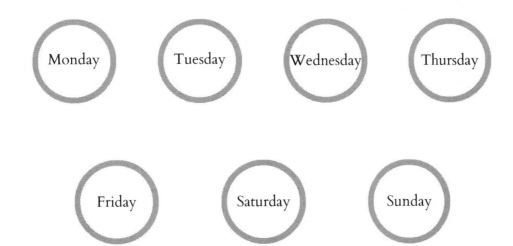

Monday   Tuesday   Wednesday   Thursday

Friday   Saturday   Sunday

Personal Pronoun

Look at the picture and circle the correct pronoun.

(boy)	He She It	(dog)	He She It
(bee)	He She It	(girl)	He She It
(table)	He She It	(woman)	He She It
(cherries)	He She It	(bicycle)	He She It

Community Helpers

Connect the pictures on the left side with their right occupation.

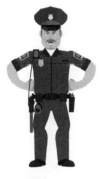 •

• doctor

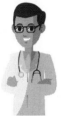 •

• engineer

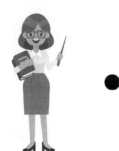 •

• fireman

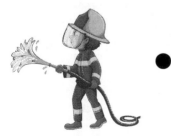 •

• police

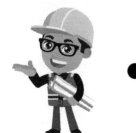 •

• teacher

Beginning Sounds

Circle the letter that each picture starts with.

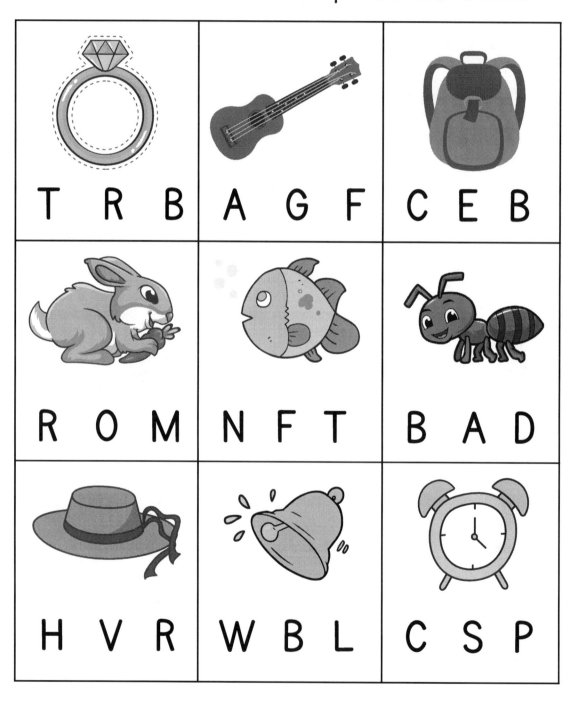

T R B   A G F   C E B

R O M   N F T   B A D

H V R   W B L   C S P

Animals

Direction: Circle the correct animal picture.

bird	
monkey	
rabbit	
lion	
cow	
pig	

Identify the pictures on the blue column. Can you tell where they get their energy from? Circle the correct answer.

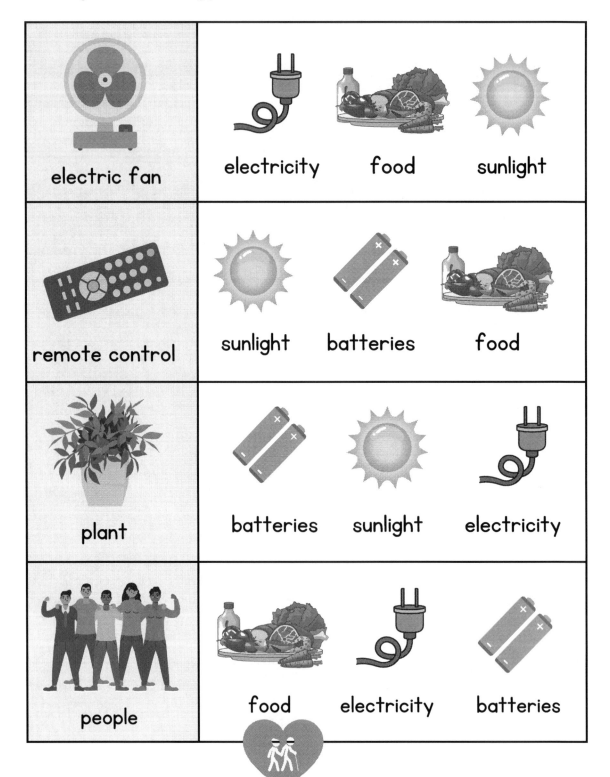

electric fan	electricity	food	sunlight
remote control	sunlight	batteries	food
plant	batteries	sunlight	electricity
people	food	electricity	batteries

Healthy and Unhealthy Food

Direction: Circle the healthy foods.

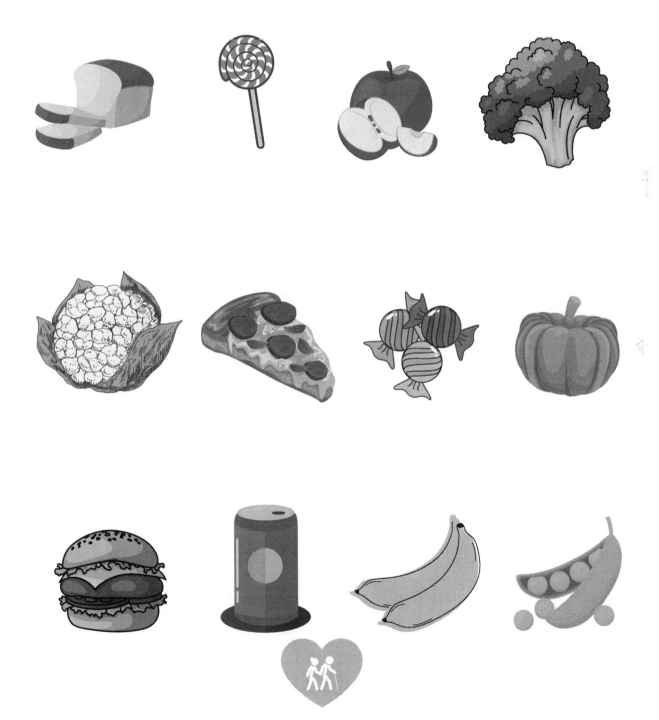

Sides of Geometric Shapes

Circle the number of sides each shape has.

Trapezoid	5	2	4
Square	6	4	2
Triangle	3	2	6
Circle	10	0	1

Opposite Words

Draw a line to match each picture with its opposite.

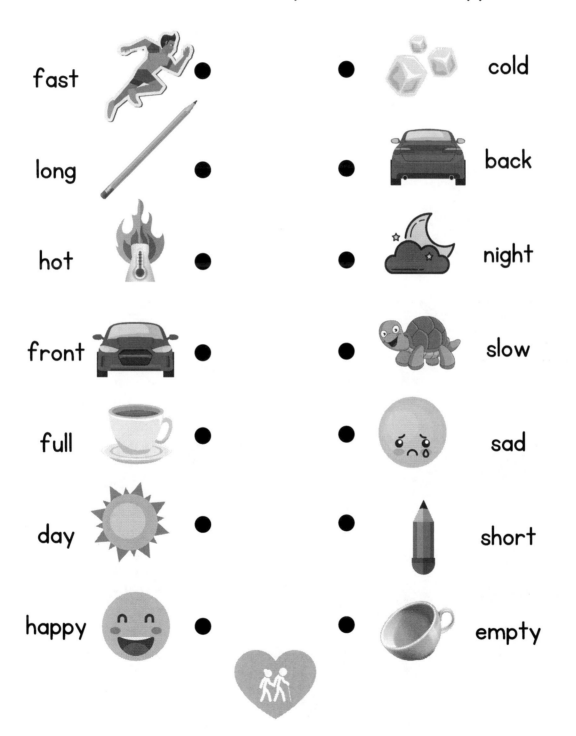

fast

long

hot

front

full

day

happy

cold

back

night

slow

sad

short

empty

Identify and match each computer term.

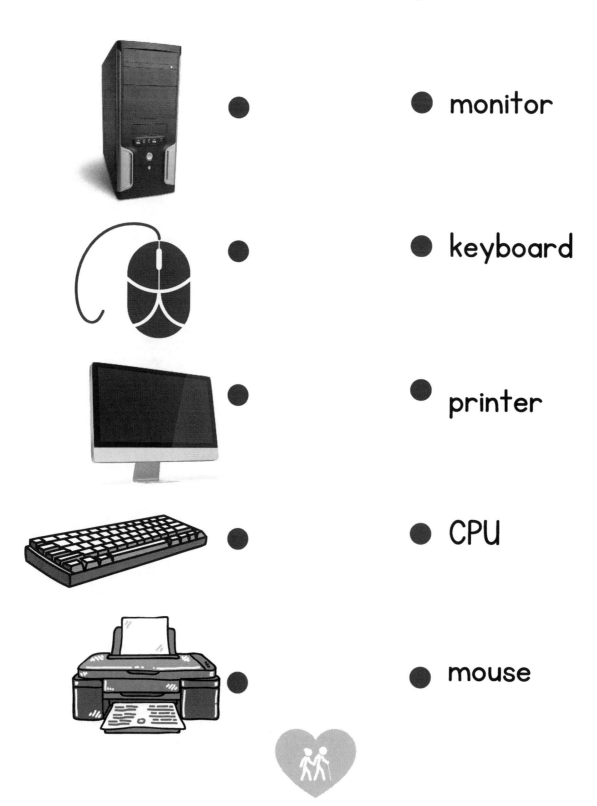

Look at the pictures below. Cut and paste them into the correct box.

pets	not pets

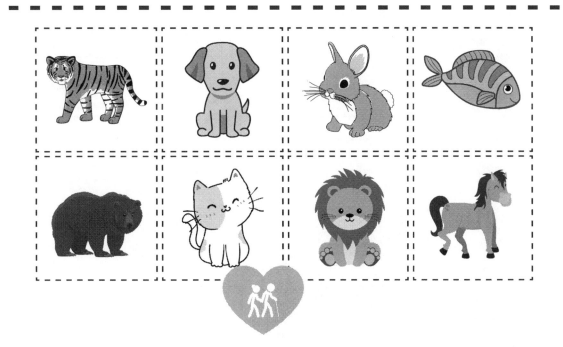

Look at the picture and circle the correct word.

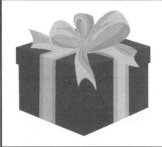

present

gift

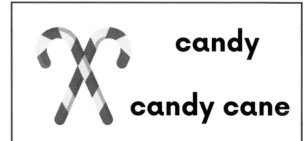

candy

candy cane

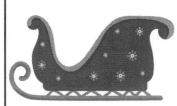

sleigh

slay

star

holly

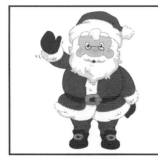

santa

elf

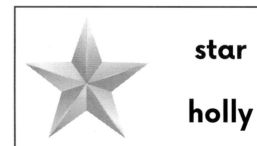

elf

santa

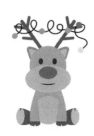

raindeer

reindeer

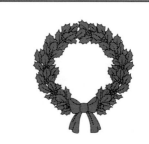

wreath

star

Find the Difference

Circle the picture that is different from the group.

1.)

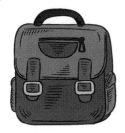 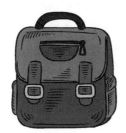 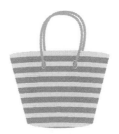 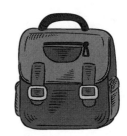

2.)

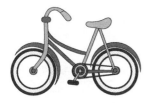 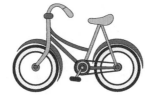 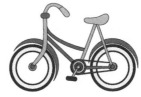 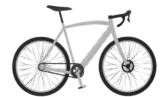

3.)

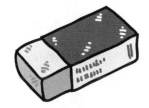 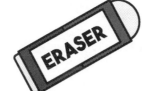 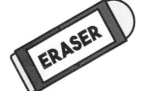 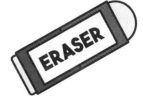

4.)

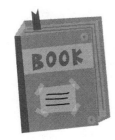 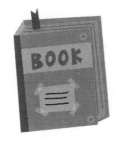 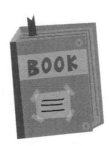 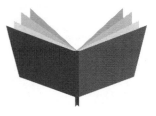

Farm or Zoo Animal

Cut and paste the pictures in the correct box.

Farm Animal	Zoo Animal

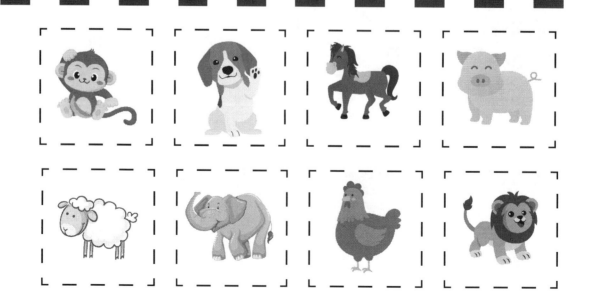

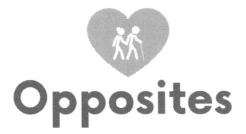

Opposites

Match the pictures which are opposites.

happy

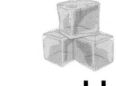

cold

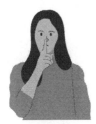

quite

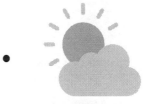

day

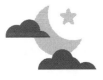

night

noisy

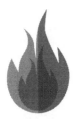

hot

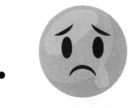

sad

Time of the Day

Match the time of the day to the correct picture.

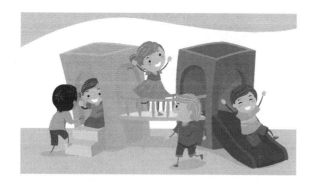

morning

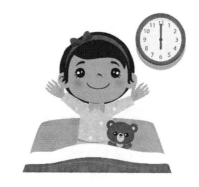

afternoon

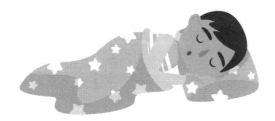

evening

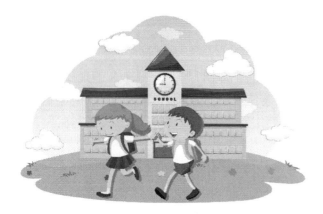

night

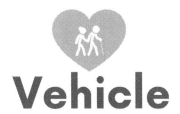

Vehicle

Match the vehicle with its name.

•   • **ship**

•   • **sailboat**

•   • **rowboat**

•   • **submarine**

Color the letters.

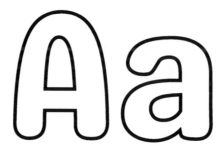

Write the letters.

A

a

Aa

Color the things that starts with Aa.

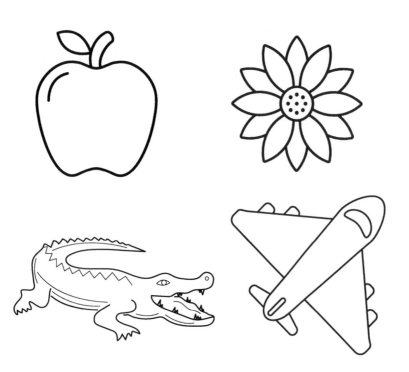

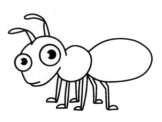

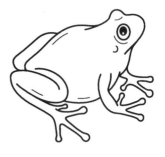

Color the letters.

B b

Write the letters.

B

b

Bb

Color the things that starts with Bb.

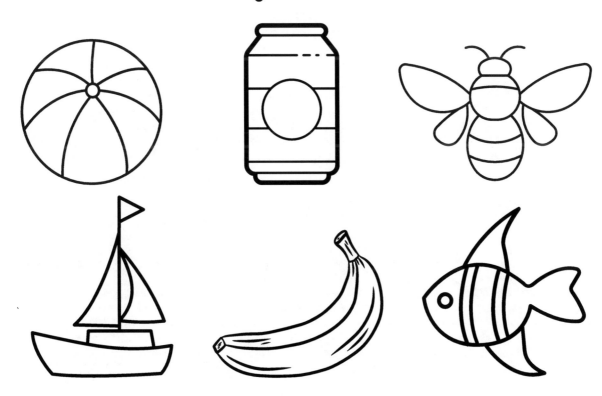

Color the letters.

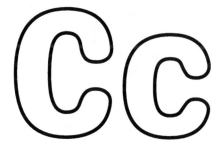

Write the letters.

C

c

Cc

Color the things that starts with Cc.

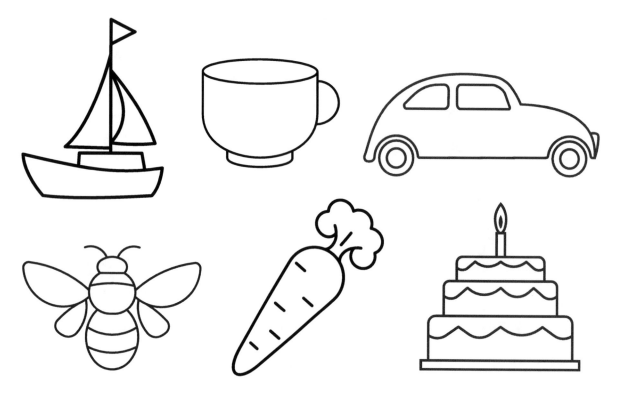

A and An

Direction: Complete each sentence with the best article.

1. It is ___ egg.

2. It is ___ car.

3. It is ___ bear.

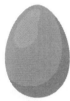 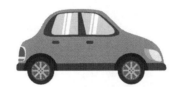 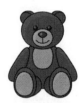

4. It is ___ elephant.

5. It is ___ apple

6. It is ___ ball.

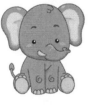 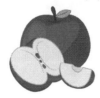

7. It is ___ ant.

8. It is ___ bike.

9. It is ___ igloo.

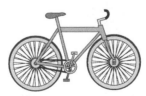 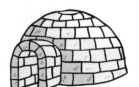

Action Words

Study the given pictures and write the appropriate action words.

dancing	eating	walking
reading	jumping	singing

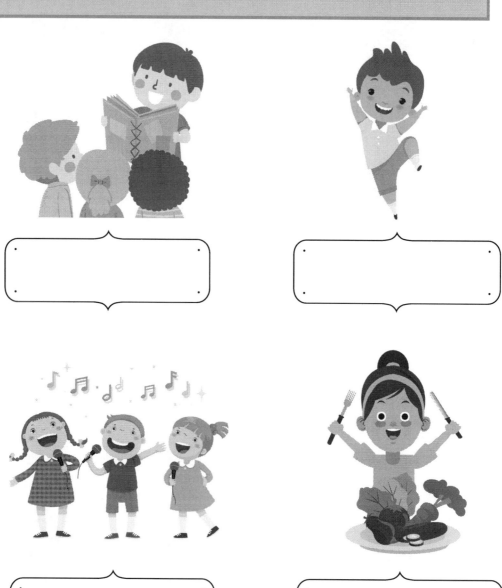

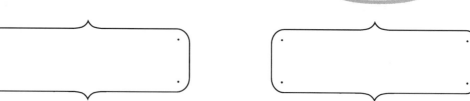

Jumbled Words

Figure out what the word is and write it on the blank provided.

g t a o	t h a n p l e e	k e y m o n
_____	_____	_____
s e r r a e	k o o b s	b g a
_____	_____	_____
p p l e a	m o n l e	o a r g e n
_____	_____	_____

Tracing the Letter Ee

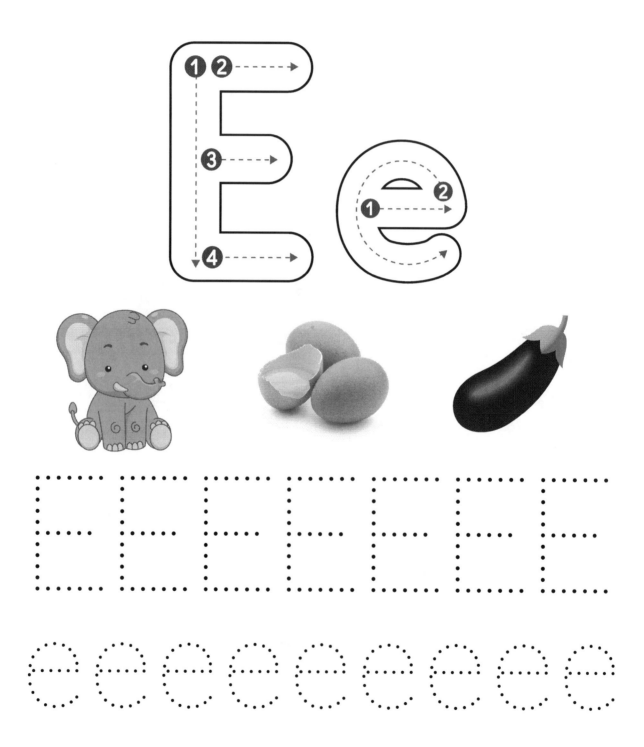

Let's Count!

Direction: Circle the correct number of images.

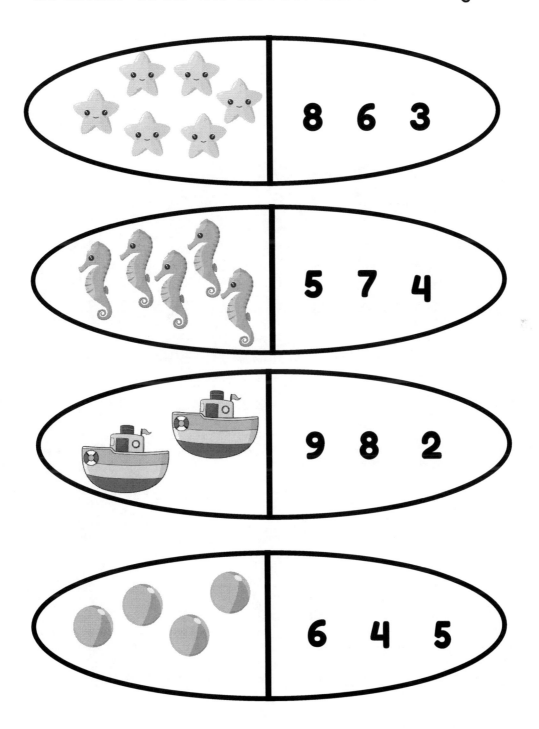

8   6   3

5   7   4

9   8   2

6   4   5

Line of Symmetry

Draw a line to divide these shapes in half evenly.

Example:

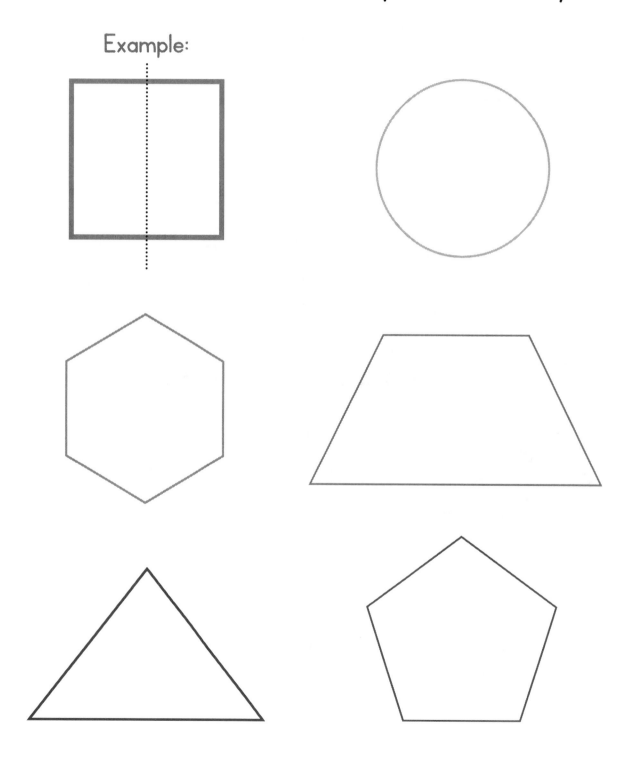

Letter P p

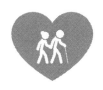

Trace the words that starts with letter P.

pan

pie

pencil

pig

Ordinal Numbers

Write <u>1st</u>, <u>2nd</u>, <u>3rd</u> and <u>4th</u> under the correct picture.

Then fill in the blanks in the sentence below.

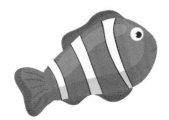 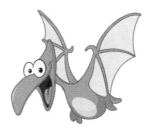 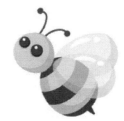 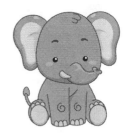

_____   _____   _____   _____

1. The is in the _____ place.

2. The is in the _____ place.

3. The is in the _____ place.

4. The is in the _____ place.

Fruit or Vegetable?

Circle the fruits. Draw a square around vegetables.

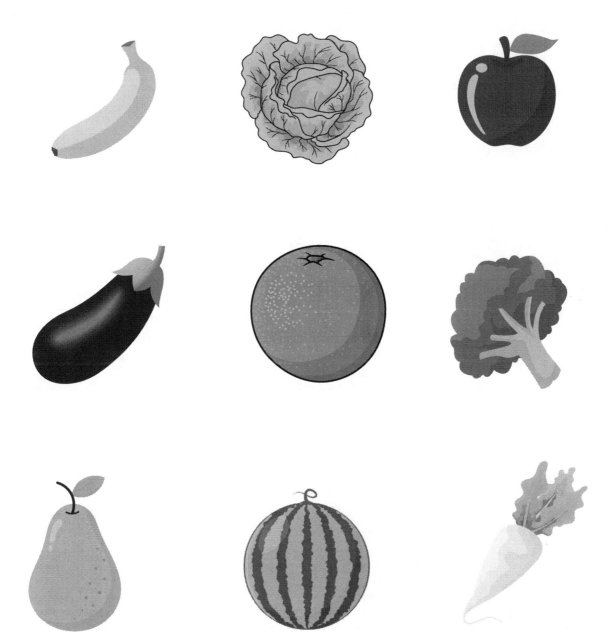

Letter Ll

Direction: Circle the pictures that start with the letter "Ll".

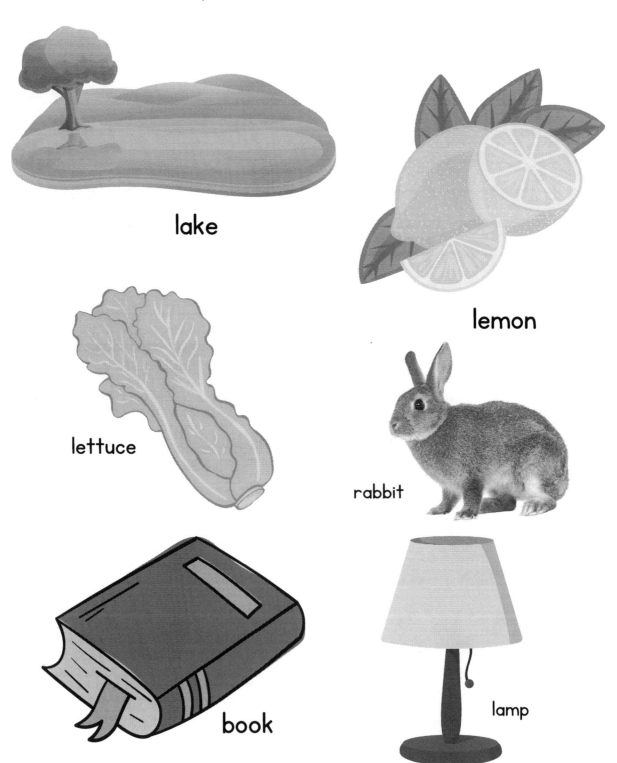

lake

lemon

lettuce

rabbit

book

lamp

Name the Vegetables

Identify each vegetables below. Choose the answer from the box.

cauliflower	red pepper	garlic
peas	potato	onion

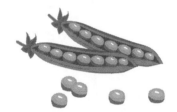   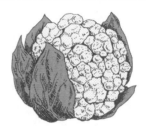

_____   _____

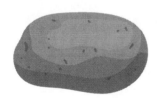   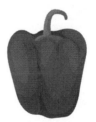

_____   _____

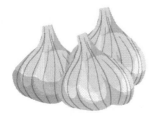   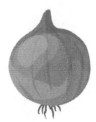

_____   _____

Name the Fruits

Identify each fruit below.

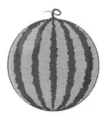

_____

_____

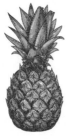

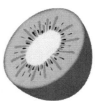

_____

_____

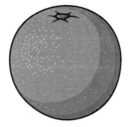

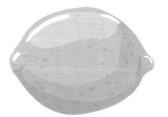

_____

_____

Beginning Blends

Please write the beginning blends to the word.

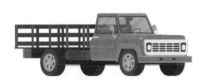

_ _ uck

_ _ ar

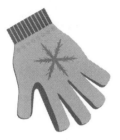

_ _ ove

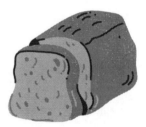

_ _ ead

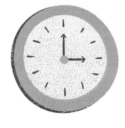

_ _ ock

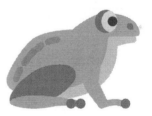

_ _ og

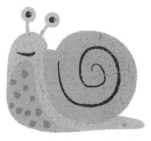

_ _ ail

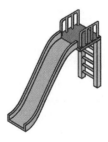

_ _ ide

Verb Tense

Use the table below to fill in the boxes to make the verb true for the correct tense of past tense, present tense, and future tense.

Yesterday I	I am	Tomorrow I will
Jumped	Jumping	Jump
Walked		Walk
	Sitting	
		Skip
Danced		
	Watching	

Articles

An article is a word that comes before a noun. Use one of the two articles to agree with the nouns below.

A   An

	_____cat
	_____egg
	_____mouse
	_____ostrich
	_____book
	_____arm
	_____ant
	_____leaf

Synonyms and antonyms

Look at each word in the first column. Circle their synonyms and cross out their antonyms.

| Tiny | Little | Huge | Large |

| Wrong | Correct | False | Good |

| Over | Under | Below | Above |

| Easy | Hard | Simple | Tough |

| End | Start | Begin | Finish |

Fill in the blanks using "ing" in its correct form.

1. The bird is _____ (flying / flew) in the sky.

2. The baby is _____ (crying / cried) because he is hungry.

3. The cat is _____ (purring / purred) on the bed.

4. The children are _____ (playing / played) in the park.

5. The dog is _____ (barking / barked) at the mailman.

6. The fish is _____ (swimming / swam) in the pond.

7. The horse is _____ (galloping / galloped) in the field.

8. The kids are _____ (laughing / laughed) at the funny joke.

9. The leaves are _____ (falling / fell) from the tree.

10. The monkey is _____ (swinging / swung) from the branch.

11. The rabbit is _____ (hopping / hopped) in the garden.

12. The turtle is _____ (crawling / crawled) on the ground.

13. The water is _____ (flowing / flowed) down the river.

14. The wind is _____ (blowing / blew) through the trees.

15. The worker is _____ (building / built) a house.

GRAMMAR ADVENTURE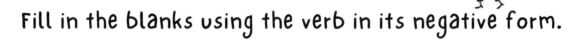

Fill in the blanks using the verb in its negative form.

1. The boy _____ (isn't / doesn't) swimming in the pool.

2. The flowers _____ (aren't / don't) blooming in winter.

3. The cat _____ (isn't / doesn't) chasing the mouse.

4. The bird _____ (isn't / do) singing in the morning.

5. The dogs _____ (aren't / don't) barking at the visitors.

6. The children _____ (aren't / don't) playing outside today.

7. The teacher _____ (isn't / doesn't) teaching the lesson.

8. The train _____ (isn't / doesn't) leaving the station yet.

9. The trees _____ (aren't / are) losing their leaves in summer.

10. The baby _____ (isn't / doesn't) sleeping through the night.

11. The car _____ (isn't / is) running properly at the moment.

12. The river _____ (isn't / doesn't) flowing very fast today.

13. The snow _____ (isn't / do) falling in the middle of summer.

14. The worker _____ (isn't / are) building the house anymore.

15. The kite _____ (isn't / am) flying high in the sky today.

Fill in the blanks using the verb in its correct form.

1. _____ the dog barking at the postman? (Is / Are)

2. _____ the children playing in the playground? (Is / Are)

3. _____ the baby crying in the crib? (Is / Are)

4. _____ the bird flying in the sky? (Is / Are)

5. _____ the cat sleeping on the couch? (Is / Are)

6. _____ the rabbit hopping in the garden? (Is / Are)

7. _____ the flowers blooming in the spring? (Is / Are)

8. _____ the monkey swinging from the tree? (Is / Are)

9. _____ the workers building the new house? (Is / Are)

10. _____ the river flowing swiftly today? (Is / Are)

11. _____ the wind blowing through the trees loudly? (Is / Are)

12. _____ the teacher explaining the lesson clearly? (Is / Are)

13. _____ the car running smoothly on the road? (Is / Are)

14. _____ the snow falling gently from the sky? (Is / Are)

15. _____ the leaves changing colors in the fall? (Is / Are)

OPPOSITE ADJECTIVES

Young – happy – sad – short – open – small – old – tall – closed– big

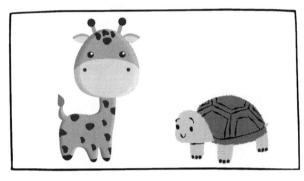

_____ X _____

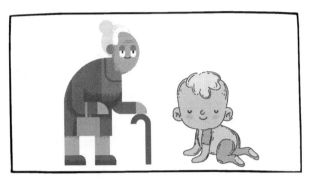

_____ X _____

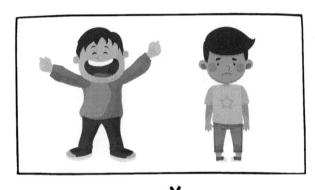

_____ X _____

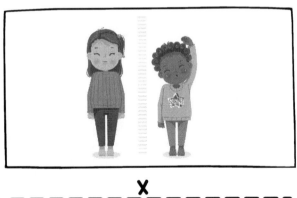

_____ X _____

X

_____

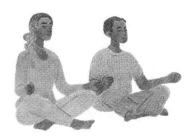

Present Continuous: What are they doing?
Look at the pictures and write sentences. Use the present continuous tense.

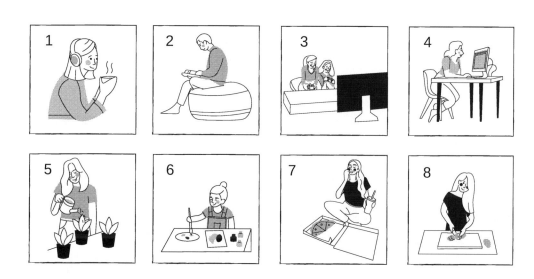

1- She's listening to music.

2- ....

3- ....

4- ....

5- ....

6- ....

7- ....

8- ....

The Power of E

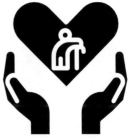

Adding an e to the end of a one syllable word makes the vowel before it say its name. This is called a magic e. Look at the example below.

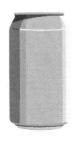

can

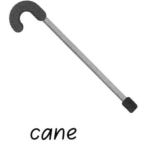

cane

Write each of the words on the lines below.

_____

- -

_____

What are these items? Write the names below.

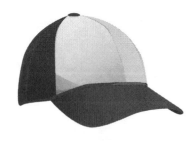

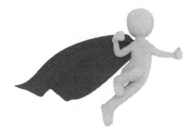

_____

- -

_____

 # ch Blends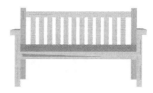

Please add a ch to each of the following letters below to
create a new word. Read the new word out loud.

su   mu   lat

ri   hat   cat

ben   lun   pat

in   op   ase

ip   ick   oke

Read the short story below and draw a picture of what is happening.

We sat on the bench to eat lunch. The rich cake and punch were good!

Christmas Syllables

Color and count the syllables in the Christmas vocabulary below.

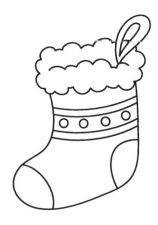

stocking

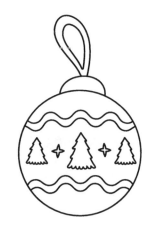

ornament

 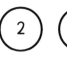

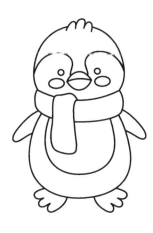

penguin

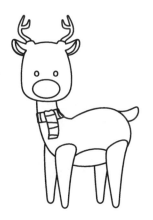

reindeer

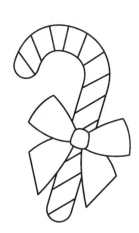

candy cane

snowman

ALL ABOUT MY NAME

My name is:

My name has the letters:

(Color the letters of your name.)

A B C D E F G H I J
K L M N O P Q R
S T U V W X Y Z

My name has:

◯ letters   ◯ syllables

My name means:

SYLLABLE SORT

A syllable is made up of vowels and/or consonants. It must contain at least one vowel sound made by an a, e, i, o, u or y or a blend of vowels.

Sort the words based on the number of syllables they contain by dragging them into the right box.

1 SYLLABLE	2 SYLLABLES	3 SYLLABLES	4 SYLLABLES
		fantastic	

pasta   calculator   begun   another

ice   one   after   make

toilet   change   avocado   house

Tanka Poem

Tanka means 'short song' and is an ancient Japanese form of poetry that tells a story of life, feelings or nature. Modern Tanka poems are broken into five poetic lines. The basic structure of a tanka poem is 5 – 7 – 5 – 7 – 7. Tankas contain different types of literary devices, such as personification, metaphors, & similes.

EXAMPLE: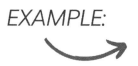

SPRINGTIME

Cherry blossoms swirl

sweetly scenting the air with

brand new beginnings.

Each petal whispers softly

as it sashays: Spring is here.

Your Turn

1. _____	5 syllables
2. _____	7 syllables
3. _____	5 syllables
4. _____	7 syllables
5. _____	7 syllables

Back to School Labyrinth

Help the little girl to grab her backpack.

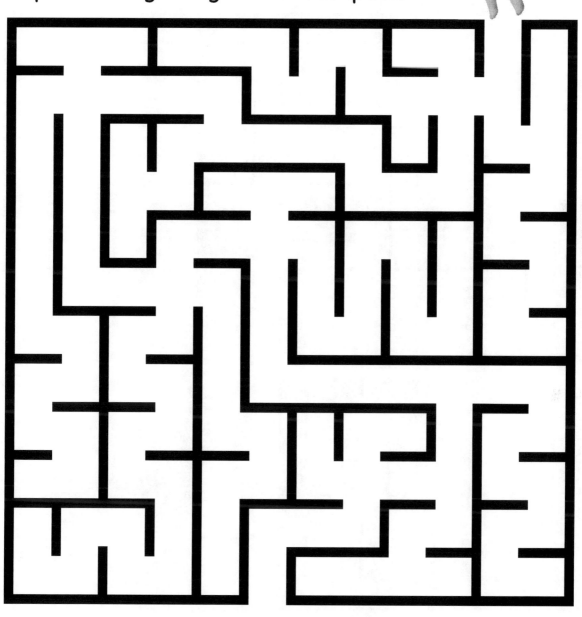

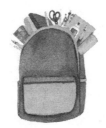

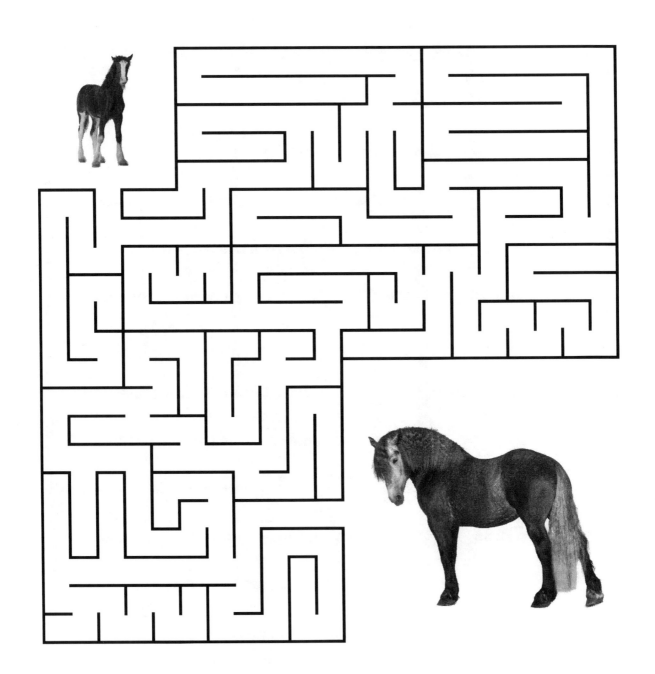

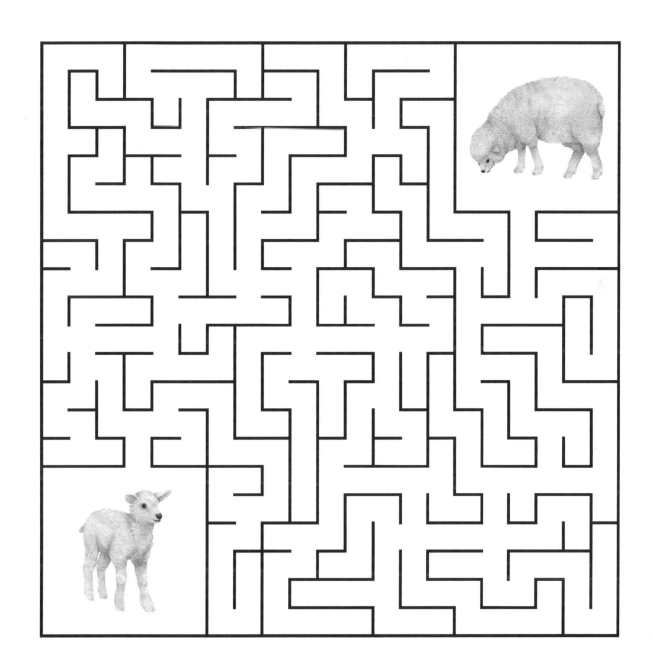

Q IS FOR...

Follow the guide to trace the letters, then complete the mazes:

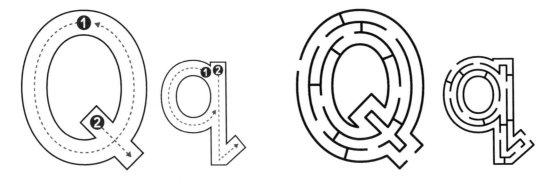

Practice writing the letters on the lines below:

------------------------------------   ------------------------------------   ------------------------------------

_____   _____   _____

_____   _____   _____

------------------------------------   ------------------------------------   ------------------------------------

Draw three things that begin with the letter Q:

Colour only the items that begin with the letter Q:

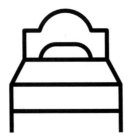  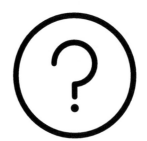

S IS FOR...

Follow the guide to trace the letters, then complete the mazes:

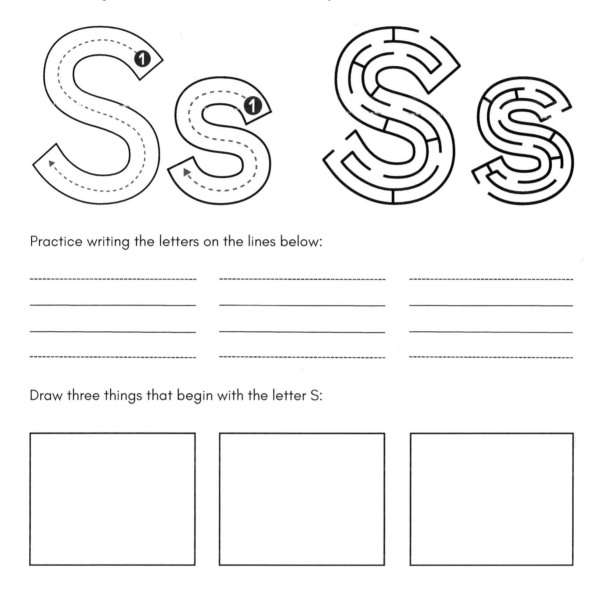

Practice writing the letters on the lines below:

----------------------------------   ----------------------------------   ----------------------------------

_____   _____   _____

_____   _____   _____

----------------------------------   ----------------------------------   ----------------------------------

Draw three things that begin with the letter S:

Colour only the items that begin with the letter S:

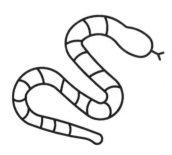  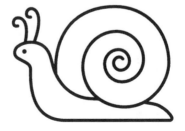

T IS FOR...

Follow the guide to trace the letters, then complete the mazes:

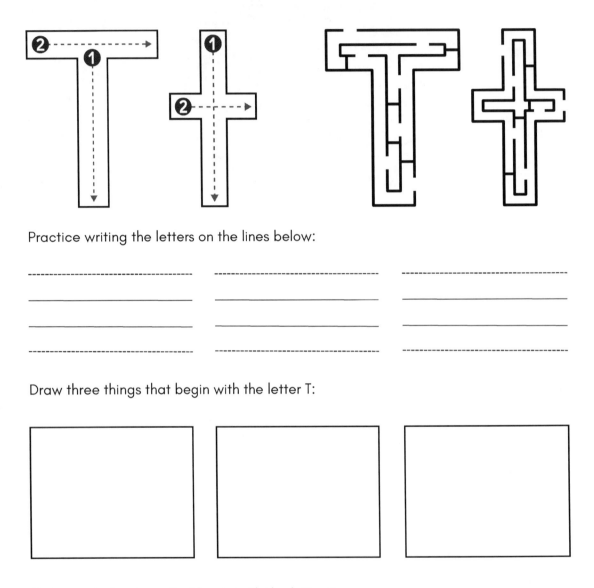

Practice writing the letters on the lines below:

------------------------------ ------------------------------ ------------------------------

_____ _____ _____

_____ _____ _____

------------------------------ ------------------------------ ------------------------------

Draw three things that begin with the letter T:

Colour only the items that begin with the letter T:

C IS FOR...

Follow the guide to trace the letters, then complete the mazes:

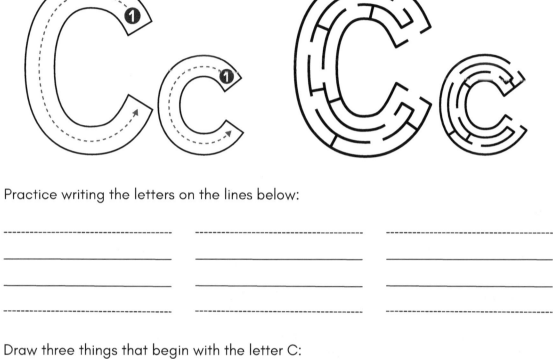

Practice writing the letters on the lines below:

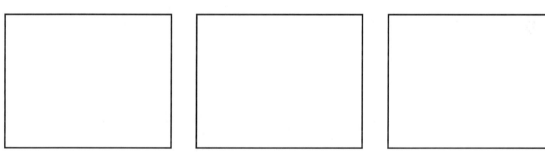

Draw three things that begin with the letter C:

Colour only the items that begin with the letter C:

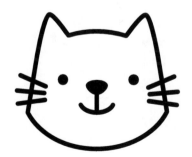 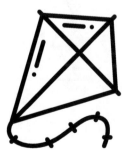 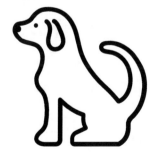

J IS FOR...

Follow the guide to trace the letters, then complete the mazes:

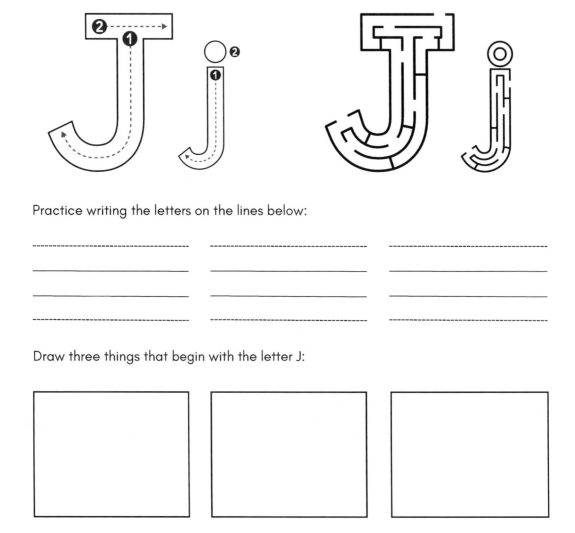

Practice writing the letters on the lines below:

------------------------------------   ------------------------------------   ------------------------------------
_____   _____   _____
_____   _____   _____
------------------------------------   ------------------------------------   ------------------------------------

Draw three things that begin with the letter J:

Colour only the items that begin with the letter J:

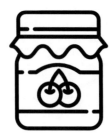

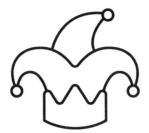

D IS FOR...

Follow the guide to trace the letters, then complete the mazes:

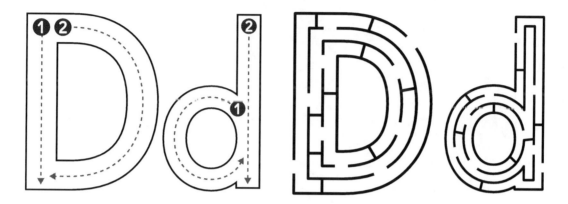

Practice writing the letters on the lines below:

------------------------------------   ------------------------------------   ------------------------------------

_____   _____   _____

_____   _____   _____

------------------------------------   ------------------------------------   ------------------------------------

Draw three things that begin with the letter D:

Colour only the items that begin with the letter D:

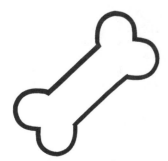
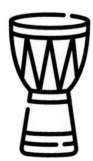
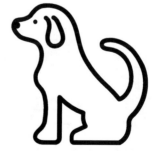

Mandala Coloring

Mandala Coloring

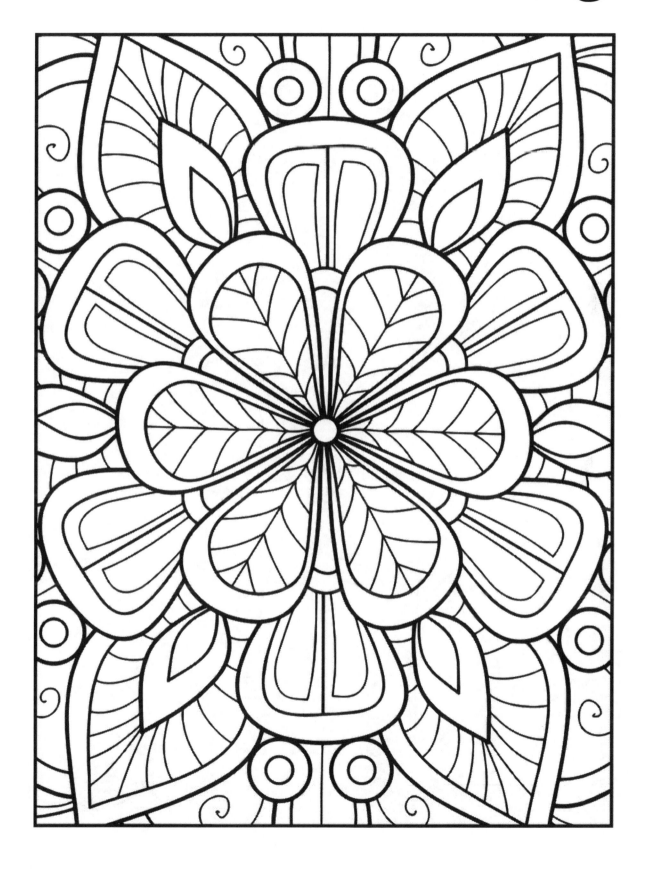

Mandala Coloring

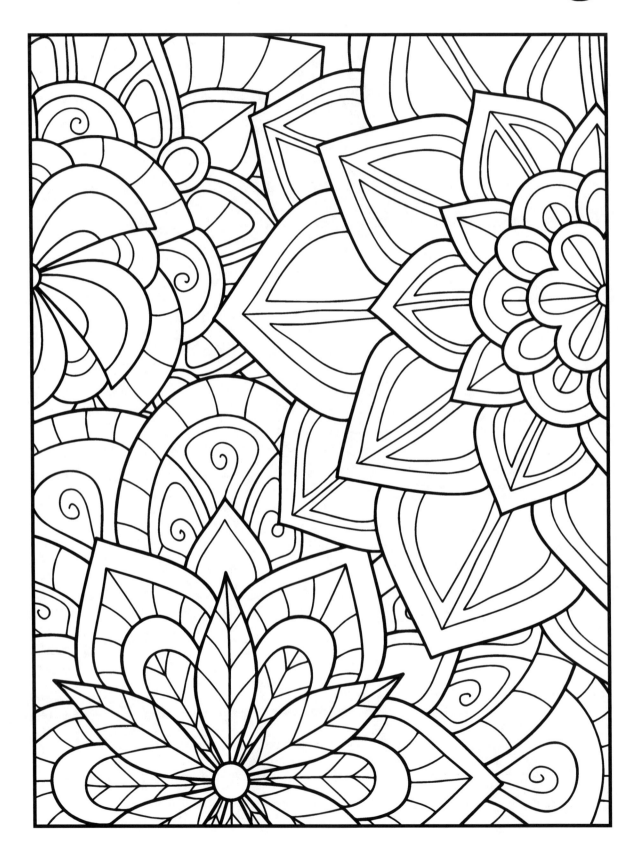

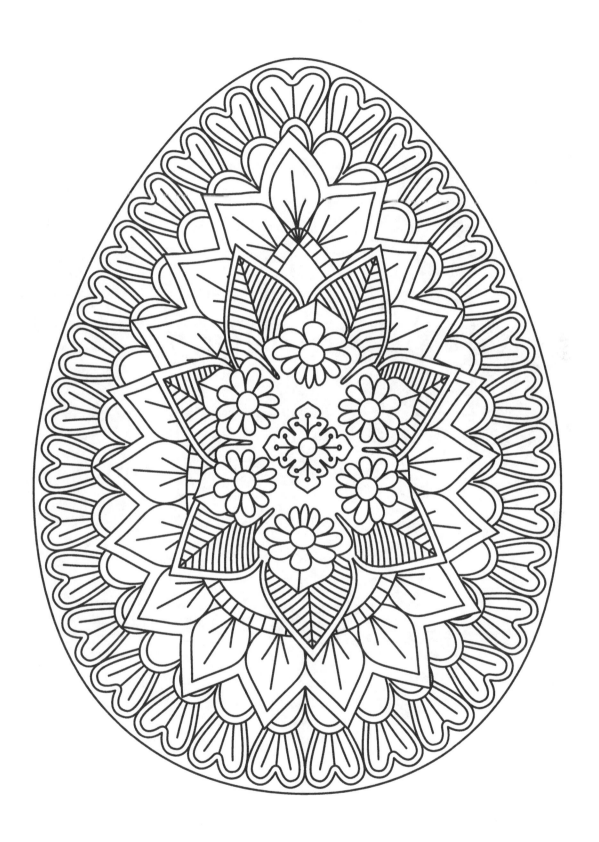

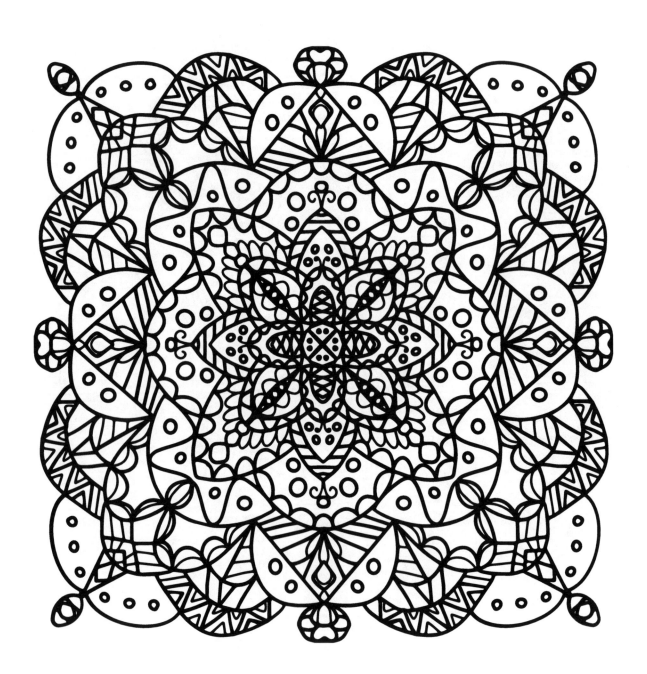

Rhyming Words

Draw a line to connect the two rhyming words.

cat	Pam
leg	blue
mad	mit
dim	fad
box	hat
fit	Tim
log	fox
Sue	keg
ham	dog

Flamingo Rhyming Practice

Circle the words that rhyme with the word on the flamingo.

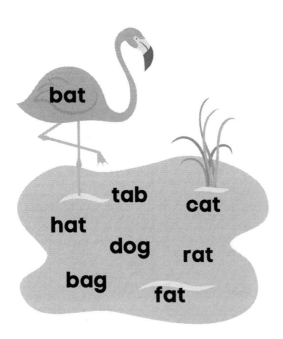

bat

tab
cat
hat
dog
rat
bag
fat

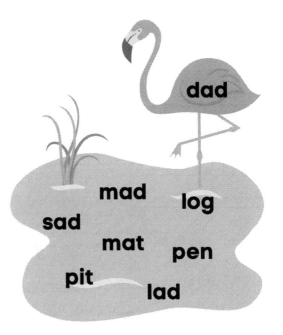

dad

mad
log
sad
mat
pen
pit
lad

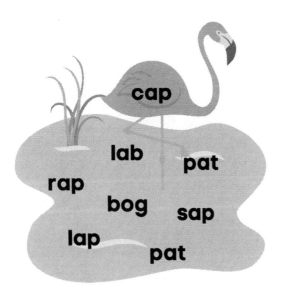

cap

lab
pat
rap
bog
sap
lap
pat

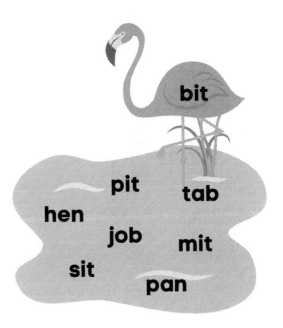

bit

pit
tab
hen
job
mit
sit
pan

Rhyming Words

Circle the word that rhymes
with the word inside the box.

cat	bat	clap
pan	saw	can
bee	see	me
hand	land	bend
mop	lap	cop
lip	skip	drip

English Rhyming Words

Directions: Circle the word that rhymes with the word on the left.

Great	Bread	Plate	Dead
Speak	Leak	Crate	Fake
Tell	Girl	Limp	Sell
Hand	Man	Land	Barn
Grow	More	Far	Flow
Wrap	Trap	Path	Lamp
Far	Shore	War	Door

Colour the images in each row that rhyme when read out loud:

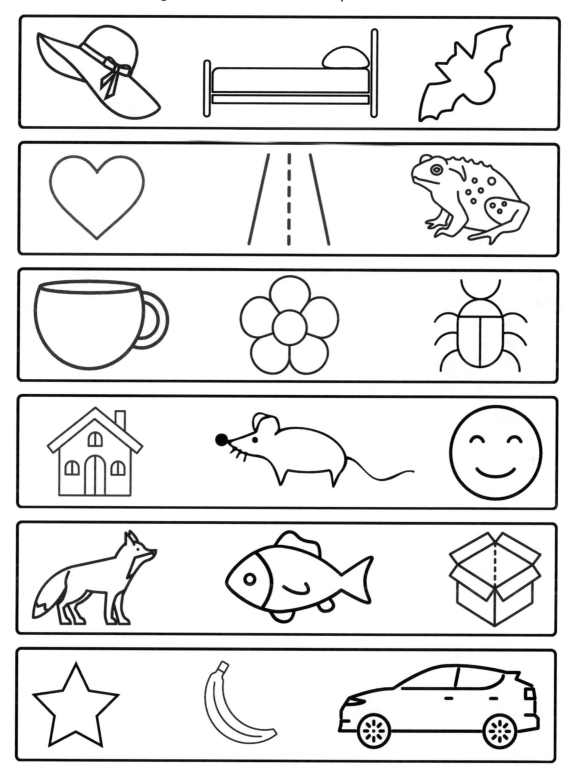

Count and Color

Count the objects and color the correct number.

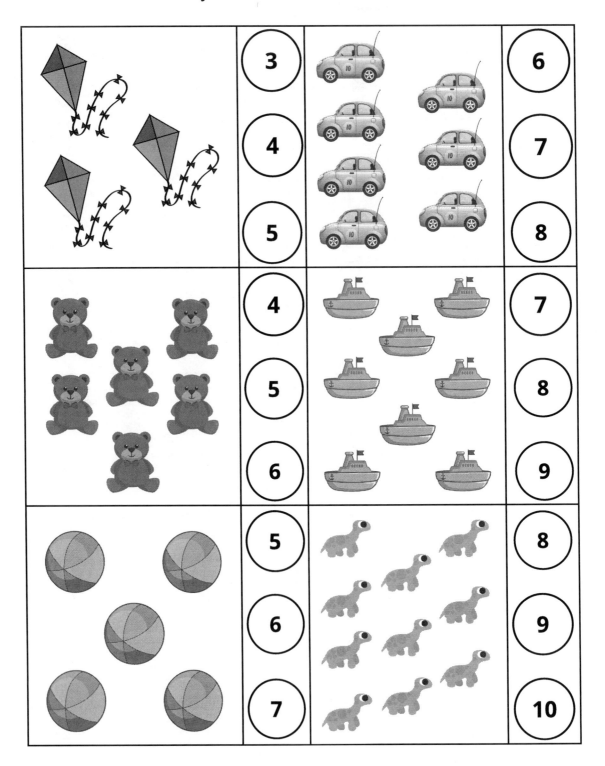

Count the number of each item and write the number in the box.

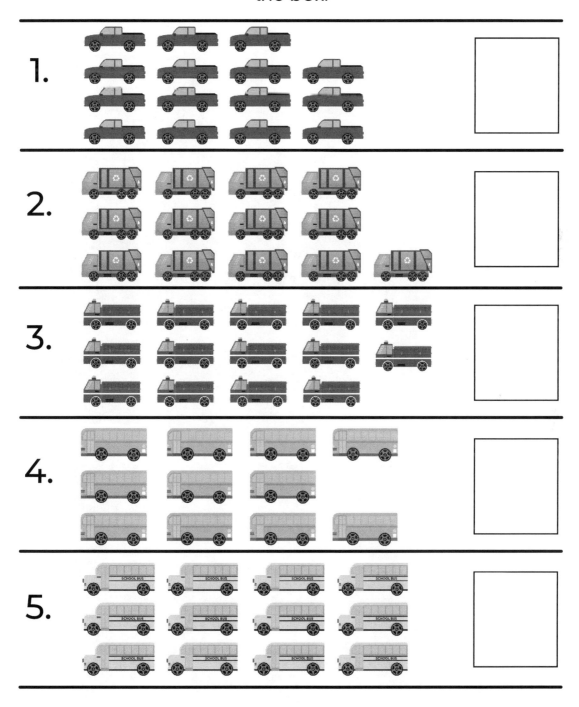

1.

2.

3.

4.

5.

NUMBER SENSE

Connect each dice to its matching numeral and popsicle sticks.

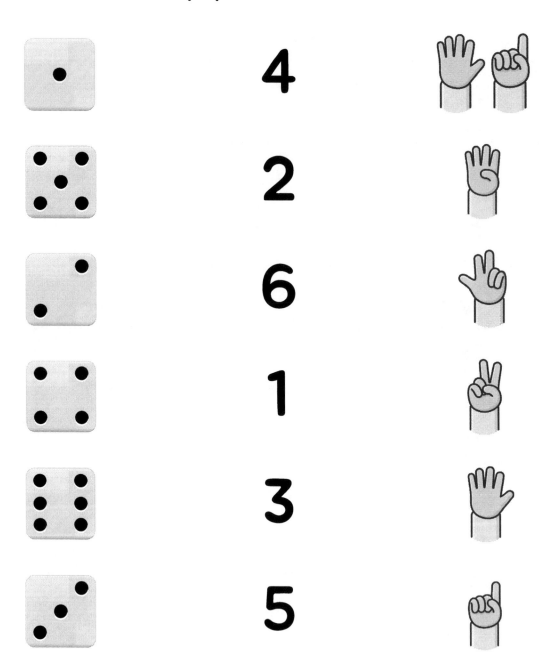

- **Write one less.**

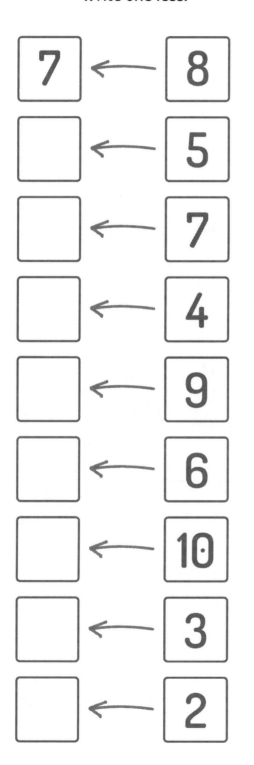

7	←	8
	←	5
	←	7
	←	4
	←	9
	←	6
	←	10
	←	3
	←	2

- **Write in increments of 1.**

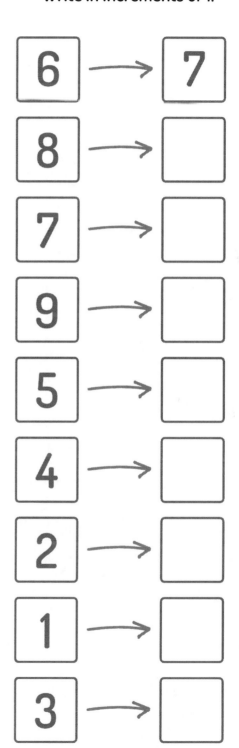

6	→	7
8	→	
7	→	
9	→	
5	→	
4	→	
2	→	
1	→	
3	→	

Cut the numbers at the bottom of this page. Count by fives by pasting the missing numbers in the boxes to complete the sequence.

5		15	20	
	35	40		50
55		65	70	
80			95	

45	90	75	85	30
100	40	25	10	60

How many?

Observe and count the shapes. Answer the questions.

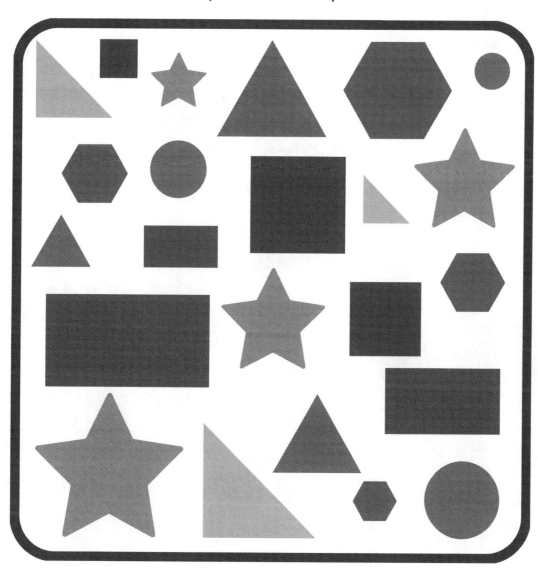

1. How many are red? ....
2. How many are small? ....
3. How many are triangle? ....
4. How many are four-sided? ....
5. How many have more than four side? ....
6. How many stars are there? ....

How many? - Key

Observe and count the shapes. Answer the questions.

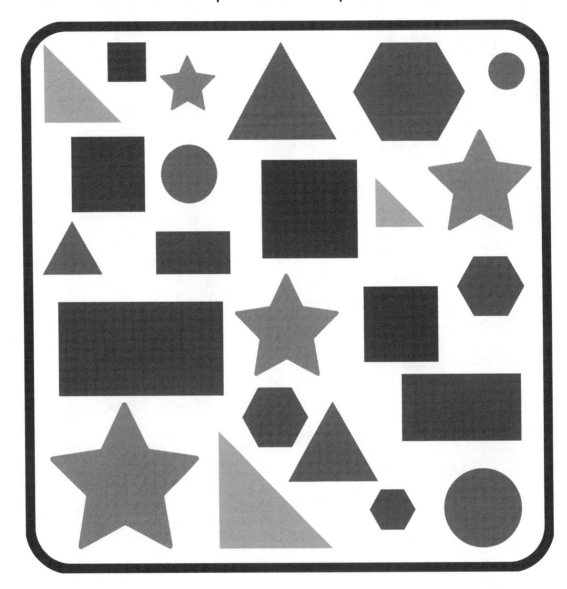

1. How many are red? ....3.................
2. How many are small? ....5.................
3. How many are triangle? ....6.................
4. How many are four-sided? ....7.................
5. How many have more than four side? ....4.................
6. How many stars are there? ....4.................

I SPY: VEGETABLES

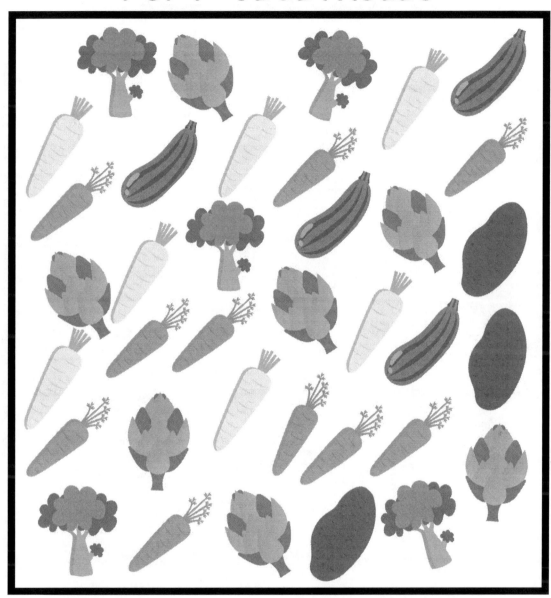

Find and count the following vegetables.

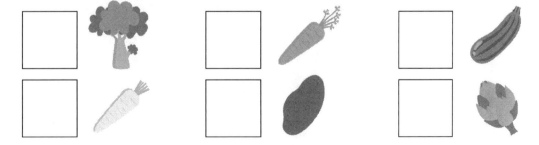

Count and Write

How many shapes are there? Count and write.

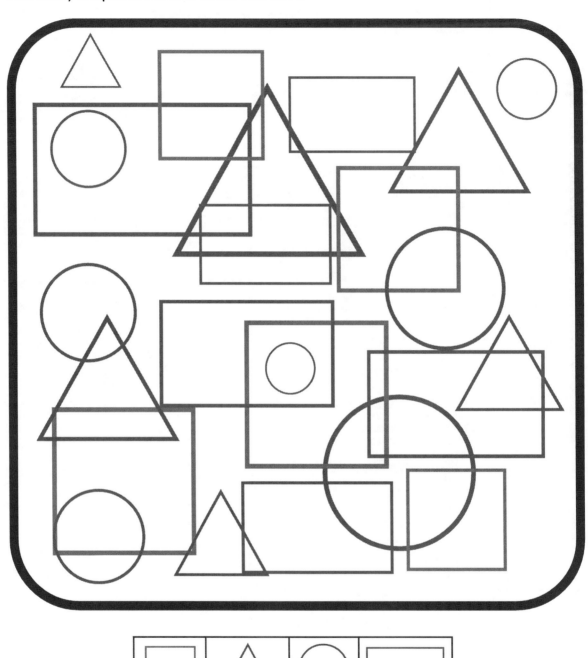

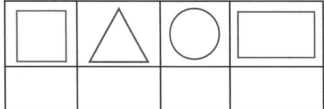

Count and Write - Key

How many shapes are there? Count and write.

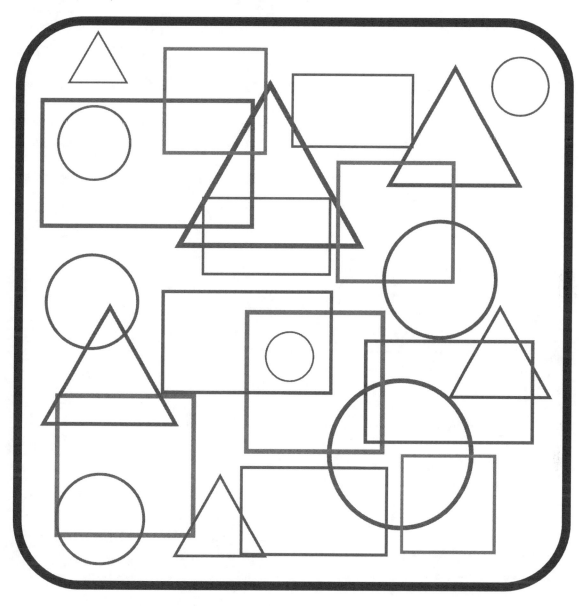

☐	△	◯	▭
5	6	7	6

COUNT TO 100

Fill in the missing numbers and count to 100.

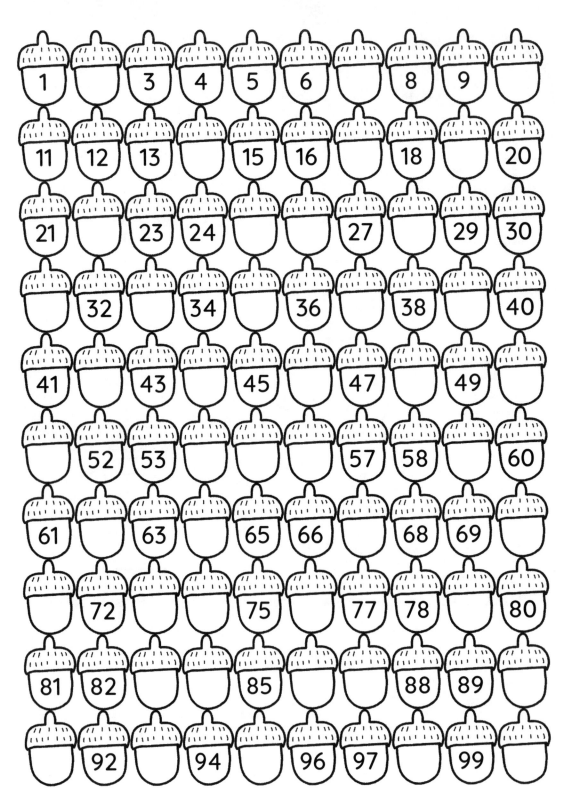

1		3	4	5	6		8	9	
11	12	13		15	16		18		20
21		23	24			27		29	30
	32		34		36		38		40
41		43		45		47		49	
	52	53				57	58		60
61		63		65	66		68	69	
	72			75		77	78		80
81	82			85			88	89	
	92		94		96	97		99	

ANIMAL PHONICS

Color the correct beginning sound of the following pictures.

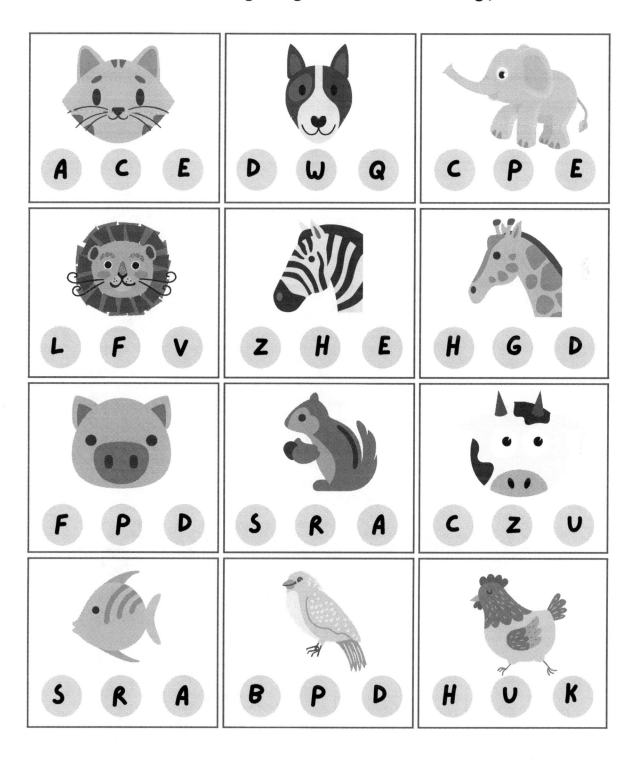

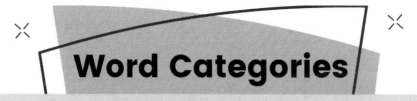

Word Categories

Move the words below into the correct boxes for nouns, adjectives, and verbs.

house	happy	grow	cat
sad	car	doctor	drink
fast	blue	eat	round
school	fly	funny	hot

Noun	Verb	Adjective
_____	_____	_____
_____	_____	_____
_____	_____	_____
_____	_____	_____
_____	_____	_____

Create a sentence using two of the words above:

_____

_____

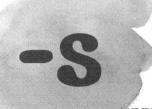

-s

Classify plural words and third person verbs according to -s pronunciation

books	dishes	hats	prizes
boxes	works	watches	babies
plays	dreams	sleeps	sisters

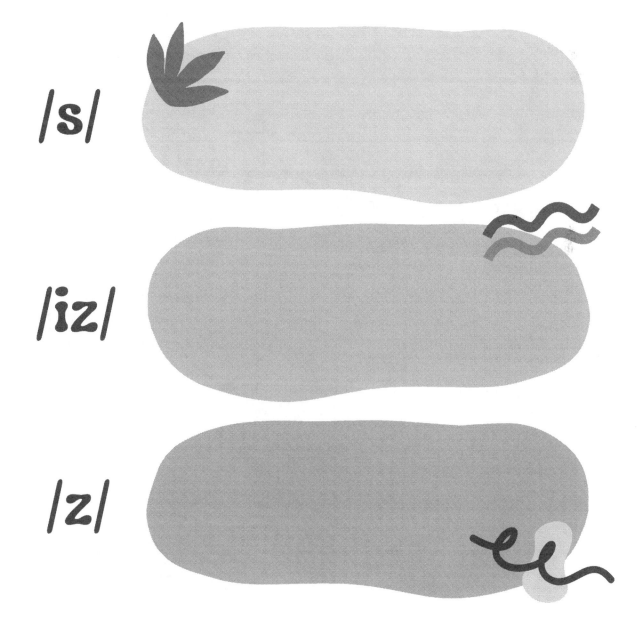

|s|

|iz|

|z|

RHYME
TIME

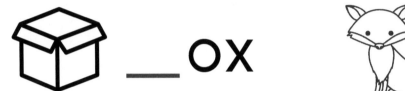 __ox   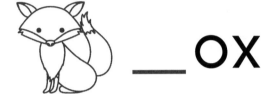 __ox

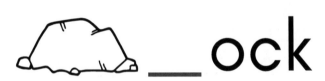 __ock   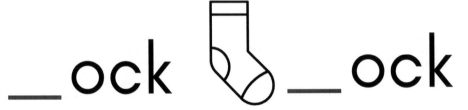 __ock

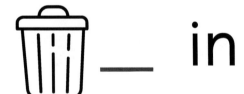 __ in   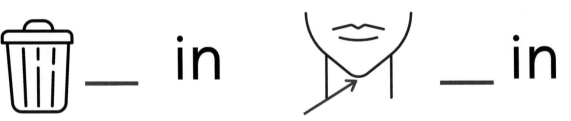 __ in

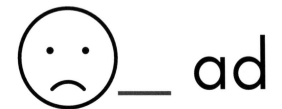 __ad   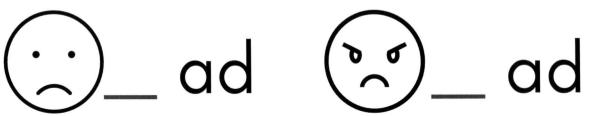 __ad

English Rhyming Words

Directions: Circle the word that rhymes with the word on the left.

Great	Bread	Plate	Dead
Speak	Leak	Crate	Fake
Tell	Girl	Limp	Sell
Hand	Man	Land	Barn
Grow	More	Far	Flow
Wrap	Trap	Path	Lamp
Far	Shore	War	Door

Christmas Spelling

Color and write the correct letter that has the beginning sound of each word.

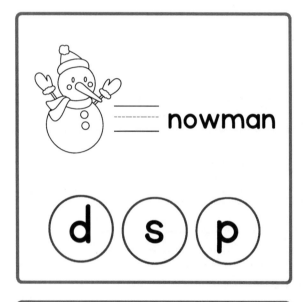 _____ nowman

d   s   p

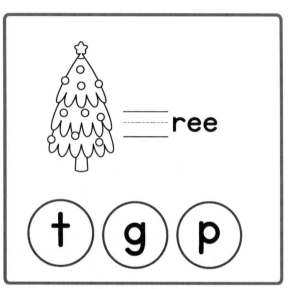 _____ ree

t   g   p

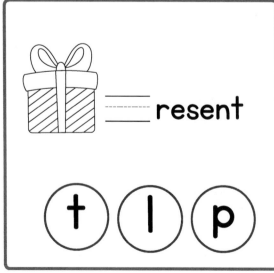 _____ resent

t   l   p

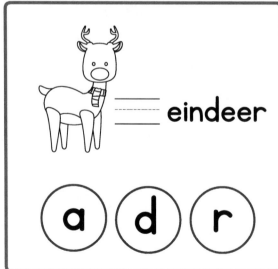 _____ eindeer

a   d   r

Rhyming WORDS

Instructions: Read out loud the written word. The picture next to each word represents something that rhymes with the word. Spell the rhyming word.

1 Mat ___ ___ ___

2 Ban ___ ___ ___

3 Run ___ ___ ___

4 Car ___ ___ ___

5 Bag ___ ___ ___ ___

6 Stand ___ ___ ___ ___

7 Sing ___ ___ ___ ___

8 Cram ___ ___ ___ ___

SUMMER WORD SEARCH

Look for the words listed below.

```
S U N W A N P U A
U S B A E I P L H
N H T T W C L S O
B E N E U E A A T
L L W R R D Y N N
O L N B O T S D F
C A M B E A C H U
K U W A V E S C N
P I N E A P P L E
```

Sun   Waves   Fun   Pineapple
Sunblock   Hot   Beach   Water
Play   Sand   Shell   Umbrella

LETTER MIX-UP!

Unscramble the letters to spell the words correctly

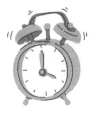 c k l c o

_ _ _ _ _

 o l b e g

_ _ _ _ _

 a t p e

_ _ _ _

 s o e s h

_ _ _ _ _

 n t a i p

_ _ _ _ _

 a l e d m

_ _ _ _ _

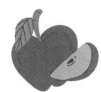 p l p e a

_ _ _ _ _

 s i p n

_ _ _ _

EMOTIONS

WORD SEARCH

Find the words listed below and mark them.

D	E	A	E	X	C	I	T	E	D	A	S
C	O	N	F	U	S	E	D	Y	E	D	U
A	B	G	O	T	U	V	S	Z	N	F	R
U	F	R	U	S	T	R	A	T	E	D	P
P	G	Y	H	C	I	J	D	I	R	H	R
S	K	O	L	A	S	U	V	R	V	A	I
E	P	M	U	R	A	T	I	E	O	P	S
T	N	Q	R	E	W	O	Y	D	U	P	E
B	O	R	E	D	U	Z	E	D	S	Y	D

- HAPPY
- SAD
- CONFUSED
- FRUSTRATED
- BORED
- NERVOUS
- SURPRISED
- UPSET
- SCARED
- ANGRY
- EXCITED
- TIRED

PLACES IN TOWN

Match the things with the places listed below.

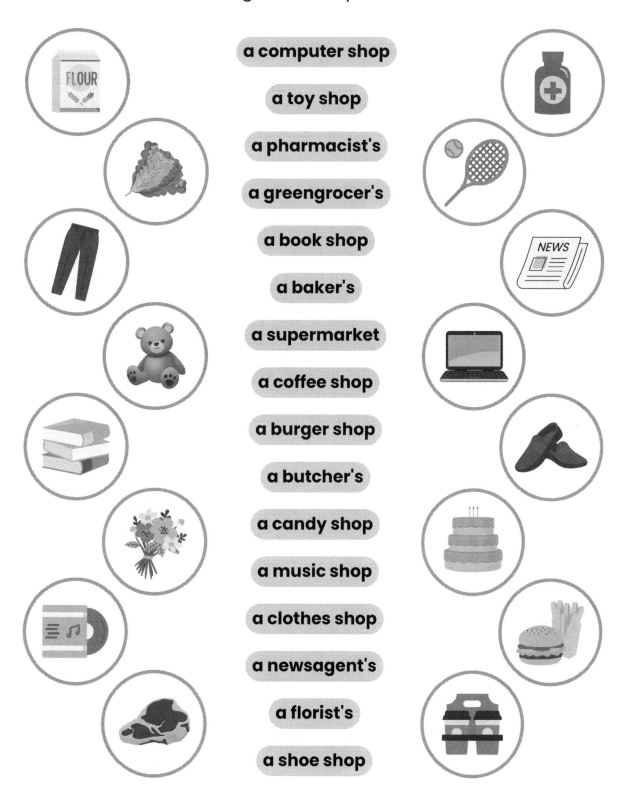

a computer shop

a toy shop

a pharmacist's

a greengrocer's

a book shop

a baker's

a supermarket

a coffee shop

a burger shop

a butcher's

a candy shop

a music shop

a clothes shop

a newsagent's

a florist's

a shoe shop

LETTER MIX-UP!

Unscramble the letters to spell the words correctly

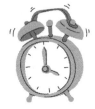 c k l c o

_ _ _ _ _

 o l b e g

_ _ _ _ _

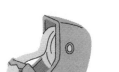 a t p e

_ _ _ _

 s o e s h

_ _ _ _ _

 n t a i p

_ _ _ _ _

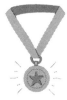 a l e d m

_ _ _ _ _

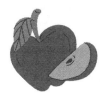 p l p e a

_ _ _ _ _

 s i p n

_ _ _ _

SYLLABLE SORT

A syllable is made up of vowels and/or consonants. It must contain at least one vowel sound made by an a, e, i, o, u or y or a blend of vowels.

Sort the words based on the number of syllables they contain by dragging them into the right box.

1 SYLLABLE	2 SYLLABLES	3 SYLLABLES	4 SYLLABLES
		fantastic	

pasta   calculator   begun   another

ice   one   after   make

toilet   change   avocado   house

Beginning Blends

Please write the beginning blends to the word.

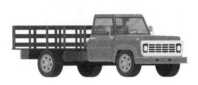

_ _ uck

_ _ ar

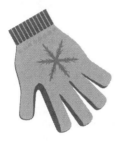

_ _ ove

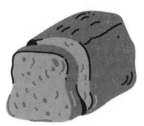

_ _ ead

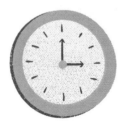

_ _ ock

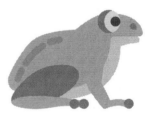

_ _ og

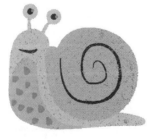

_ _ ail

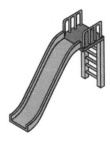

_ _ ide

Phonics: Mm

Trace using 5 colors on each: Complete the puzzles:

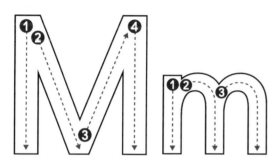 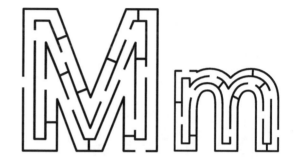

Practice correct letter formation for Mm:

_____

- -

- -

_____

Brainstorm words that use each of these sounds:

/ m /
map

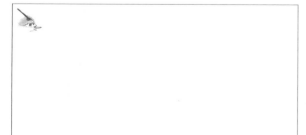

Read these 'm' words:

mix

mat

map

mug

mom

Sentence Correcting

Rewrite the sentences in the space provided. Make sure to use capital letters, proper spelling, and punctuation.

1. i see the cat

_____

2. do you see the fish

_____

3. it's time for lunch

_____

4. what color is your hat

_____

5. the dog is barking

_____

What am I?

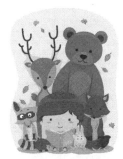

Directions: Start with the number one and connect the dots to find out what woodland creature I am! When finished unscramble the letters below to fill in the blank to identify me. If time permits color me.

C O O C N A R

_____ _____ _____ _____ _____ _____ _____

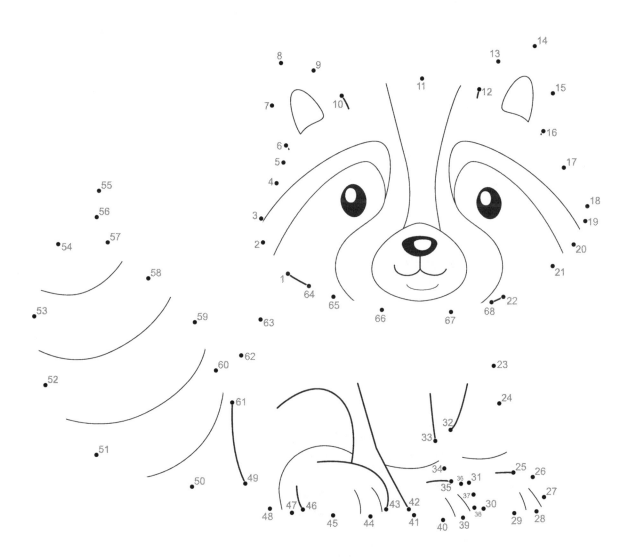

WHAT AM I?

Astronauts use me to get to their destination, what am I? Connect the dots starting with 1 to find out. When finished color me.

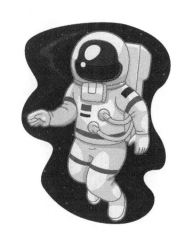

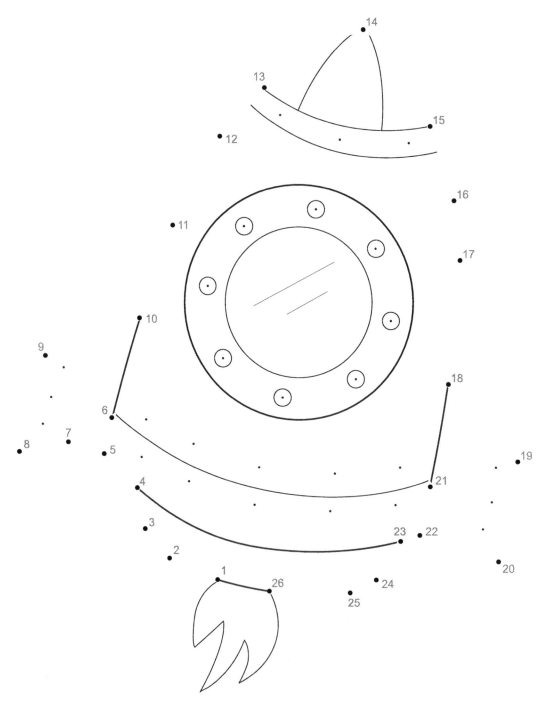

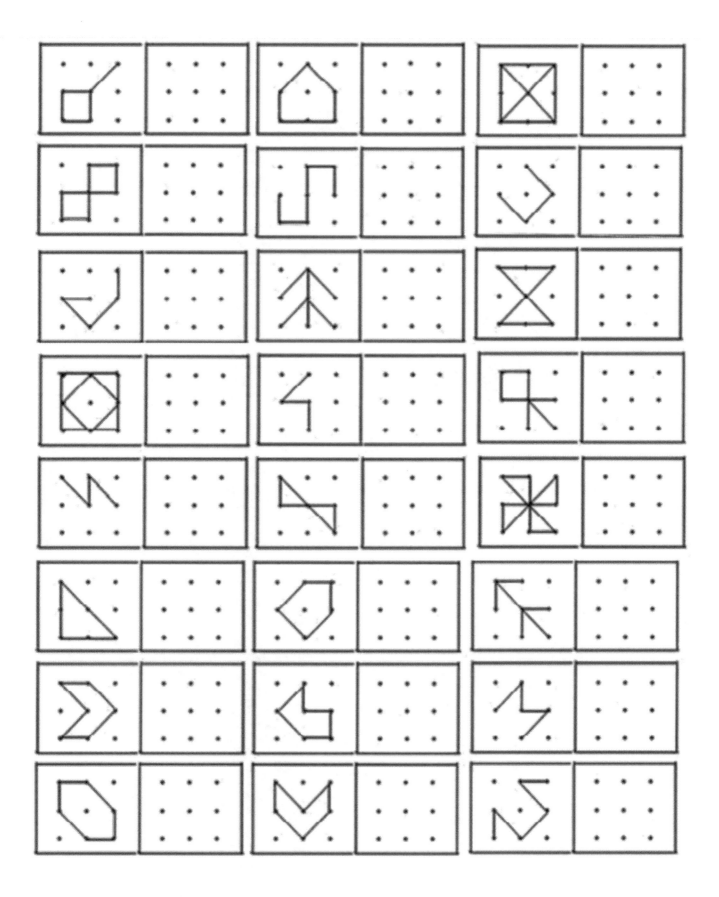

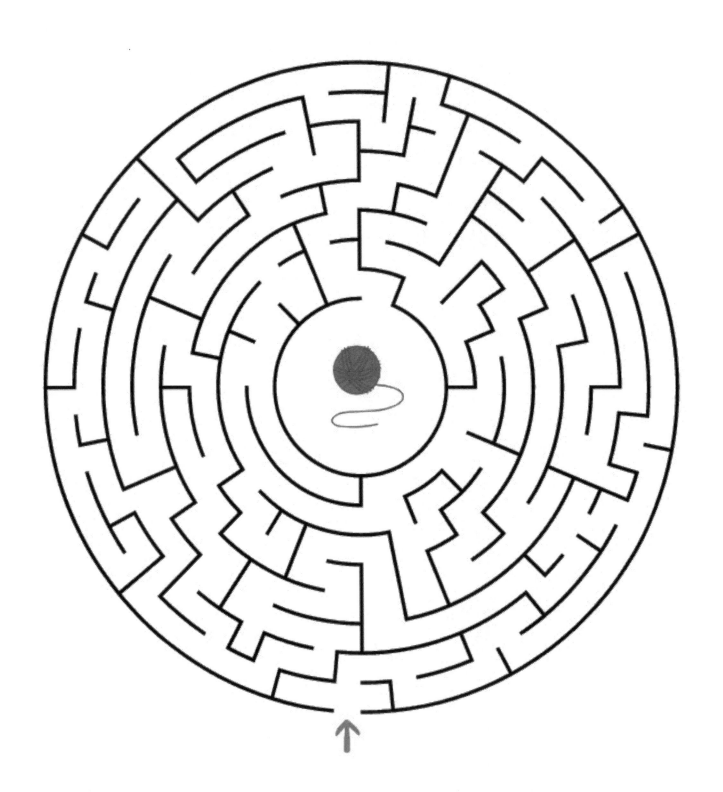

Look at the pictures and write sentences. Use the present continuous tense.

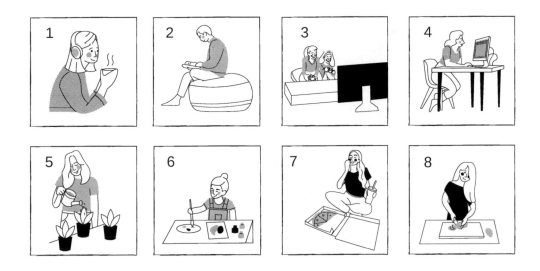

1- She's listening to music.

2- ....

3- ....

4- ....

5- ....

6- ....

7- ....

8- ....

Made in the USA
Middletown, DE
17 October 2023

40975585R00073